OPTIMAL HEALTH:

ACHIEVING BALANCE THROUGH FITNESS AND WELLNESS

In our fast-paced modern world, maintaining optimal health and fitness has become more crucial than ever. "Achieving Wellness: A Comprehensive Guide to Health and Fitness" is a comprehensive book designed to empower individuals on their journey to a healthier and more fulfilling life.

This book encompasses a wide range of topics, including the importance of health and fitness in today's society, setting goals and cultivating a healthy mindset, the impact of exercise on physical and mental well-being, the role of nutrition in maintaining optimal health, the significance of sleep and stress management, designing personalized workout plans, mastering nutritional balance, managing stress and emotions, integrating physical activity into everyday life, overcoming fitness plateaus and challenges, optimizing sleep and recovery, and maintaining long-term success.

With each chapter, readers will gain a deep understanding of the subject matter and discover practical strategies to implement in their own lives. The book provides valuable insights, evidence-based information, and actionable tips to help readers make sustainable changes and achieve their health and fitness goals.

Whether you are a beginner or someone seeking to enhance your current lifestyle, "Achieving Wellness" serves as a comprehensive resource, offering guidance, motivation, and support. It is a roadmap to a healthier, happier, and more vibrant you. Embark on this transformative journey and unlock your true potential for overall well-being.

DISCLAIMER:

The information provided in this book, "Optimal Living: A Comprehensive Guide to Health and Fitness," is for general informational purposes only. The content is not intended to be a substitute for professional medical advice, diagnosis, or treatment. Always seek the advice of your physician or qualified healthcare provider with any questions you may have regarding a medical condition or before starting any new fitness or dietary regimen.

The author and publisher of this book have made reasonable efforts to ensure the accuracy and completeness of the information provided. However, they make no representations or warranties of any kind, express or implied, about the suitability, reliability, or completeness of the content. The author and publisher disclaim any liability, loss, or risk incurred as a direct or indirect consequence of the use and application of any information presented in this book.

The reader should consult their healthcare provider before making any significant changes to their exercise routine, diet, or lifestyle. The author and publisher do not endorse any specific products, services, or organizations mentioned in this book unless explicitly stated.

Every individual is unique, and results may vary based on personal circumstances, commitment, and adherence to the principles and recommendations outlined in this book. The reader assumes full responsibility for their actions and decisions concerning their health and fitness journey.

By reading this book, the reader acknowledges and agrees to the above disclaimer.

TABLE OF CONTENTS

INTRODUCTION:

In today's fast-paced and demanding world, maintaining optimal health and fitness has become more crucial than ever. Our sedentary lifestyles, poor dietary choices, and increasing stress levels have led to a rise in chronic diseases and a decline in overall well-being. However, by prioritizing our health and embracing a comprehensive approach to fitness and wellness, we can regain control of our lives and achieve a state of balance.

This book, "Optimal Health: Achieving Balance through Fitness and Wellness," is designed to guide you on a transformative journey towards better health. It aims to empower you with knowledge, strategies, and practical tips to make positive changes in your lifestyle and establish sustainable habits that will enhance your physical, mental, and emotional well-being.

Setting goals and creating a healthy mindset is the first step towards achieving optimal health. By clarifying your intentions and envisioning your desired outcomes, you can cultivate the motivation and determination necessary for long-term success. This book will provide you with tools to set realistic goals, overcome self-limiting beliefs, and adopt a positive mindset that will fuel your journey towards a healthier and happier life.

Throughout the chapters that follow, you will explore the fundamental principles of health and fitness. You will gain a deeper understanding of the profound impact that exercise, nutrition, sleep, and stress management have on your overall wellness. By unraveling the complex relationship between these factors, you will learn how to harness their potential to optimize your health.

In addition to providing knowledge, this book will guide you in developing practical skills to build a solid fitness routine. You will learn how to assess your current fitness level, design a personalized workout plan, and incorporate a variety of exercises to target different aspects of physical fitness, such as cardiovascular endurance, strength, flexibility, and mobility. Whether you are a beginner or an experienced fitness enthusiast, this book will equip you with the tools necessary to create a customized exercise program that suits your individual needs and preferences.

Nutrition plays a vital role in supporting our overall health and well-being. In this book, you will delve into the foundations of nutrition, exploring the importance of macronutrients and micronutrients, and understanding how to create a balanced meal plan. You will gain insights into portion control, mindful eating, and healthy cooking techniques that will enable you to make nutritious food choices and fuel your body optimally.

However, achieving optimal health is not solely about physical fitness and nutrition. The mind-body connection is a powerful aspect of our well-being, and this book acknowledges its significance. You will discover strategies for stress management, relaxation, and mindfulness practices that can help you navigate the challenges of daily life and cultivate emotional resilience.

Integrating physical activity into our everyday lives is key to maintaining long-term health and well-being. This book will provide practical tips and guidance on how to incorporate exercise into a busy schedule, make fitness a family affair, and embrace outdoor activities to reconnect with nature's restorative powers.

While embarking on a health and fitness journey, it's essential to be prepared for challenges and setbacks. This book will equip you with strategies to overcome plateaus, stay motivated, and seek professional guidance when needed. It will also emphasize the importance of recovery and quality sleep in optimizing your overall well-being.

Ultimately, this book aims to empower you to maintain long-term success by offering strategies for consistency, setting realistic expectations, and creating a support system. It encourages you to embrace a holistic approach to health and fitness that encompasses not only physical well-being but also mental, emotional, and spiritual aspects.

Are you ready to embark on this transformative journey towards optimal health and well-being? Let's dive into the following chapters and equip ourselves with the knowledge and tools to create a healthier, more vibrant life.

The importance of health and fitness in modern society

The importance of health and fitness in modern society cannot be overstated. As we navigate the challenges of our fast-paced, technology-driven lives, it is crucial to prioritize our well-being to ensure a high quality of life and longevity. Here are some key aspects to consider:

Physical Well-being: Regular exercise and physical activity are essential for maintaining optimal physical health. Engaging in activities that promote cardiovascular endurance, strength, flexibility, and balance helps to prevent chronic diseases such as obesity, heart disease, and diabetes. Physical fitness also enhances energy levels, improves posture, and promotes healthy weight management.

Mental Health: The impact of physical fitness on mental health is profound. Exercise stimulates the release of endorphins, also known as "feel-good" hormones, which boost mood, reduce stress, and alleviate symptoms of anxiety and depression. Regular physical activity has been linked to improved cognitive function, enhanced memory, and increased creativity. By prioritizing fitness, we can enhance our overall mental well-being and cultivate a positive mindset.

Productivity and Performance: In today's competitive world, being physically fit can significantly impact our productivity and performance in various domains of life. Exercise improves focus, concentration, and memory, enabling us to perform better in academic or professional settings. Moreover, regular physical activity enhances energy levels, reduces fatigue, and increases resilience, all of which contribute to higher productivity and improved performance.

Disease Prevention: Chronic diseases, such as cardiovascular diseases, type 2 diabetes, certain types of cancer, and respiratory disorders, are prevalent in modern society. Many of these conditions are preventable through lifestyle choices, with physical fitness and a healthy diet playing a crucial role. By incorporating regular exercise and maintaining a balanced diet, we can reduce the risk of developing these diseases and improve our overall health outcomes.

Longevity and Quality of Life: The pursuit of health and fitness is directly linked to longevity and an enhanced quality of life. Regular physical activity, combined with healthy lifestyle choices, can increase life expectancy, improve mobility, and reduce the risk of age-related health issues. By maintaining a strong and healthy body, we can enjoy a more vibrant and active life well into our later years.

Social Connections: Health and fitness activities often provide opportunities for social interaction and community engagement. Joining fitness classes, sports teams, or recreational clubs allows us to connect with like-minded individuals who share our interests and goals. These social connections contribute to a sense of belonging, motivation, and accountability, making our fitness journeys more enjoyable and sustainable.

Role Modeling and Influence: As members of modern society, we have the opportunity to be role models for future generations. By prioritizing health and fitness, we can inspire others to adopt healthier lifestyles, fostering a culture of well-being. Setting positive examples for our children, family, friends, and colleagues can have a ripple effect, creating a healthier society as a whole.

In summary, health and fitness are integral components of modern life. Prioritizing our well-being not only benefits us individually but also has a positive impact on our communities and society at large. By embracing a lifestyle that incorporates regular physical activity, a nutritious diet, and mindful self-care practices, we can enhance our physical and mental health, prevent diseases, and lead fulfilling lives.

Setting goals and creating a healthy mindset

Setting goals and creating a healthy mindset are crucial steps in achieving long-term success in health and fitness. They provide a solid foundation for motivation, focus, and resilience throughout your wellness journey. Let's explore these concepts further:

1. Goal Setting: Setting clear and realistic goals is essential to guide your actions and measure progress. Here are some key points to consider when setting goals:

   - Specificity: Define your goals in specific terms. For example, instead of saying, "I want to get fit," specify, "I want to be able to run a 5K in under 30 minutes."

- Measurability: Establish measurable criteria to track your progress. This allows you to objectively assess your achievements and make adjustments as needed. For instance, set a goal to increase your strength by lifting a certain weight or to decrease your body fat percentage by a specific amount.

- Attainability: Ensure that your goals are realistic and attainable within a given timeframe. Setting overly ambitious goals can lead to frustration and discouragement. Break down larger goals into smaller, manageable milestones to stay motivated and focused.

- Relevance: Ensure that your goals align with your personal values and aspirations. Identify why achieving these goals is important to you. This intrinsic motivation will drive you forward during challenging times.

- Time-bound: Set deadlines or target dates for achieving your goals. This provides a sense of urgency and accountability. Breaking your goals down into short-term, medium-term, and long-term objectives can help you stay on track.

2. Creating a Healthy Mindset: Developing a healthy mindset is fundamental to maintaining consistency, resilience, and a positive outlook. Here are key aspects to consider:

   - Self-Awareness: Cultivate self-awareness by reflecting on your thoughts, emotions, and behaviors related to health and fitness. Recognize any self-limiting beliefs or negative self-talk that may hinder your progress. Practice self-compassion and replace negative thoughts with positive affirmations.

   - Positive Reinforcement: Focus on your achievements, no matter how small, and celebrate them. Acknowledge your progress and the efforts you put in. This positive reinforcement will help boost your confidence and motivation.

   - Embrace Failure as a Learning Opportunity: Understand that setbacks and failures are a natural part of the journey towards health and fitness. Instead of viewing them as defeats, see them as learning opportunities. Analyze what went wrong, adjust your approach, and use these experiences to grow stronger and wiser.

   - Adopt a Growth Mindset: Embrace the belief that your abilities and skills can be developed through dedication, effort, and learning. A growth mindset allows you to see challenges as opportunities for growth and to persevere through obstacles.

   - Surround Yourself with Support: Seek out a supportive network of family, friends, or like-minded individuals who can offer encouragement, accountability, and guidance. Share your goals and progress with them to create a positive environment that fosters motivation and success.

- Practice Mindfulness: Incorporate mindfulness practices into your routine to cultivate present-moment awareness. Mindfulness helps you develop a deeper connection with your body, emotions, and thoughts. It can enhance self-regulation, reduce stress, and improve decision-making related to your health and fitness goals.

- Focus on Long-Term Habits: Shift your perspective from short-term results to long-term habits. Instead of chasing quick fixes or temporary changes, aim to establish sustainable lifestyle habits that support your overall well-being. This approach ensures that your mindset is focused on a lifelong journey of health and fitness.

By setting goals and cultivating a healthy mindset, you lay the groundwork for a successful and fulfilling health and fitness journey. These practices provide clarity, motivation, and resilience, helping you navigate challenges and stay committed to your well-being goals. Remember to regularly review and adjust your goals as you progress and evolve throughout your journey.

Chapter 1: Understanding the Foundations of Health and Fitness

Before embarking on a journey towards optimal health and fitness, it is essential to understand the foundational principles that underpin our well-being. In this chapter, we will delve into the fundamental aspects of health and fitness, gaining a comprehensive understanding of their significance in our lives. By exploring the intricate connections between our physical, mental, and emotional well-being, we can lay the groundwork for a holistic approach to wellness.

In this chapter, we will uncover the transformative power of exercise, the vital role of nutrition, and the importance of sleep and stress management in maintaining optimal health. By unraveling these essential components, we will equip ourselves with the knowledge necessary to make informed decisions and embrace a lifestyle that supports our overall well-being.

We will begin by exploring the impact of exercise on our physical and mental health. Regular physical activity goes beyond aesthetics; it plays a crucial role in preventing chronic diseases, improving cardiovascular health, boosting energy levels, and enhancing our mood and cognitive function. By understanding the physiological and psychological benefits of exercise, we can appreciate its value as a cornerstone of our well-being.

Next, we will delve into the realm of nutrition and its profound influence on our health and fitness. By understanding the role of macronutrients and micronutrients, we can make informed dietary choices that nourish our bodies and support optimal performance. We will explore the importance of balanced eating, portion control, and mindful consumption, allowing us to fuel our bodies effectively and achieve nutritional harmony.

Sleep and stress management are integral components of our well-being that often go overlooked. In this chapter, we will uncover the significance of quality sleep in promoting physical and mental restoration, enhancing cognitive function, and supporting our overall health. Additionally, we will explore the impact of stress on our well-being and the importance of adopting effective stress management techniques to cultivate resilience and balance.

By understanding the foundational principles of health and fitness, we will gain a comprehensive perspective on how these elements interconnect and influence our overall well-being. Armed with this knowledge, we can make informed choices, set realistic goals, and create a roadmap towards a healthier, more vibrant life.

So, let us delve into the foundations of health and fitness, equipping ourselves with the knowledge and understanding that will pave the way for a transformative journey towards optimal well-being.

The impact of exercise on physical and mental well-being

The impact of exercise on physical and mental well-being is profound and far-reaching. Engaging in regular physical activity goes beyond simply improving our physical fitness; it plays a crucial role in enhancing our overall health and promoting a positive mental state. Let's explore the various ways in which exercise influences our physical and mental well-being:

Physical Health Benefits:

a) **Cardiovascular Health:** Exercise strengthens the heart and improves cardiovascular function. It increases heart rate, promotes efficient blood circulation, and helps lower blood pressure. Regular aerobic exercise, such as jogging, swimming, or cycling, reduces the risk of cardiovascular diseases, including heart attacks, strokes, and high cholesterol levels.

b) **Weight Management:** Exercise is a key component of weight management. It helps burn calories, build lean muscle mass, and increase metabolism. By incorporating both cardiovascular exercises and strength training into our routines, we can achieve a healthy body composition and maintain a healthy weight.

c) **Bone and Muscle Health:** Weight-bearing exercises, such as weightlifting or resistance training, stimulate the growth and maintenance of bone density. This helps prevent conditions like osteoporosis and reduces the risk of fractures. Exercise also promotes muscle strength, flexibility, and coordination, enhancing overall physical performance and reducing the risk of injuries.

d) **Immune System Function:** Regular exercise boosts the immune system by improving circulation and enhancing the function of immune cells. This strengthens the body's defense against infections and reduces the risk of chronic diseases.

e) **Chronic Disease Prevention:** Exercise is a powerful preventive measure against various chronic conditions, including type 2 diabetes, certain types of cancer (such as colon and breast cancer), and metabolic disorders. It improves insulin sensitivity, regulates blood sugar levels, and reduces inflammation in the body, lowering the risk of developing these diseases.

Mental Health Benefits:

a) **Mood Enhancement:** Exercise triggers the release of endorphins, neurotransmitters that create feelings of happiness and euphoria. This natural mood enhancement can help alleviate symptoms of depression, reduce anxiety, and improve overall psychological well-being. Regular exercise has been shown to be as effective as medication and therapy in treating mild to moderate depression.

b) **Stress Reduction:** Physical activity acts as a stress reliever by reducing the production of stress hormones, such as cortisol, and increasing the production of endorphins. Exercise provides an outlet for pent-up energy and tension, promoting relaxation and mental clarity.

c) **Cognitive Function:** Exercise improves cognitive function, including memory, attention, and executive function. It increases blood flow to the brain, promotes the growth of new neurons, and enhances connectivity between different brain regions. Regular exercise has been linked to a reduced risk of cognitive decline and neurodegenerative diseases, such as Alzheimer's disease.

d) **Sleep Improvement:** Exercise has a positive impact on sleep quality and duration. It helps regulate the sleep-wake cycle and promotes deep, restorative sleep. By incorporating physical activity into our daily routine, we can improve our sleep patterns and wake up feeling more refreshed and energized.

e) **Self-Esteem and Body Image:** Regular exercise can boost self-esteem and improve body image. Achieving fitness goals, building strength and endurance, and feeling confident in our physical abilities can positively impact our perception of ourselves and promote a healthy body image.

In summary, the impact of exercise on physical and mental well-being is extensive. Regular physical activity not only improves cardiovascular health, weight management, and overall physical fitness but also enhances mood, reduces stress, improves cognitive function, and promotes better sleep. By incorporating exercise into our lives, we can reap the countless benefits it offers, fostering a healthy body and a positive, resilient mind.

The role of nutrition in maintaining optimal health

The role of nutrition in maintaining optimal health is crucial. The food we consume provides our bodies with the necessary nutrients, energy, and building blocks for growth, repair, and overall functioning. A well-balanced and nutritious diet plays a pivotal role in preventing chronic diseases, supporting our immune system, promoting physical and mental well-being, and ensuring long-term health. Let's explore the various aspects of nutrition and its impact on our overall health:

Macronutrients: Macronutrients are the major nutrients our bodies require in larger quantities. They include carbohydrates, proteins, and fats.

a) **Carbohydrates:** Carbohydrates are the primary source of energy for our bodies. They are broken down into glucose, which fuels our brain, muscles, and other organs. Complex carbohydrates, such as whole grains, fruits, and vegetables, provide fiber, vitamins, and minerals along with sustained energy. Simple carbohydrates, found in sugary foods and refined grains, provide quick bursts of energy but lack nutritional value and can lead to blood sugar imbalances.

b) **Proteins:** Proteins are essential for growth, repair, and maintenance of tissues and cells in our bodies. They are composed of amino acids, which are crucial for various functions, including enzyme production, hormone regulation, and immune system support. Good sources of protein include lean meats, poultry, fish, dairy products, legumes, nuts, and seeds.

c) **Fats:** Fats are a concentrated source of energy and play a vital role in hormone production, insulation, and cushioning of organs, and the absorption of fat-soluble vitamins. Healthy fats, such as those found in avocados, nuts, seeds, and olive oil, provide essential fatty acids and contribute to heart health. Saturated and trans fats, found in processed foods, fried foods, and fatty meats, should be consumed in moderation as they can increase the risk of cardiovascular diseases.

Micronutrients: Micronutrients are essential vitamins and minerals that our bodies need in smaller quantities but are critical for proper functioning and maintaining good health. They include vitamins (such as vitamin A, C, D, E, and B vitamins) and minerals (such as calcium, iron, magnesium, and zinc). These micronutrients are involved in various bodily processes, including immune function, bone health, energy metabolism, and nerve function. Consuming a wide variety of fruits, vegetables, whole grains, legumes, nuts, and seeds ensures an adequate intake of micronutrients.

Hydration: Hydration is often overlooked but is vital for maintaining optimal health. Water is involved in nearly every bodily function, including digestion, nutrient absorption, waste removal, and temperature regulation. It is recommended to drink an adequate amount of water throughout the day to stay hydrated and support optimal body functions. Individual water needs vary depending on factors such as activity level, climate, and overall health.

Benefits of a Balanced Diet: Maintaining a balanced and nutritious diet offers numerous health benefits:

a) **Disease Prevention:** A diet rich in fruits, vegetables, whole grains, lean proteins, and healthy fats provides essential nutrients and antioxidants that help reduce the risk of chronic diseases such as heart disease, stroke, type 2 diabetes, and certain types of cancer. For example, a diet high in fruits and vegetables is associated with a lower risk of heart disease and improved cardiovascular health.

b) **Weight Management:** A balanced diet helps maintain a healthy weight. It includes appropriate portions and a variety of foods that provide essential nutrients while controlling calorie intake. Whole foods that are nutrient-dense and high in fiber promote satiety and help regulate appetite.

c) **Energy and Performance:** Proper nutrition supports optimal energy levels and enhances physical performance. Consuming adequate carbohydrates provides the necessary fuel for exercise and daily activities. Proteins support muscle repair and growth, while healthy fats provide sustained energy and aid in nutrient absorption.

d) **Mental Well-being:** Nutrition has a significant impact on our mental health and cognitive function. A balanced diet rich in essential nutrients, such as omega-3 fatty acids, B vitamins, and antioxidants, supports brain health, memory, focus, and mood stability. On the other hand, a diet high in processed foods, refined sugars, and unhealthy fats has been linked to an increased risk of mental health disorders such as depression and anxiety.

e) **Immune System Support:** Adequate nutrition is essential for a robust immune system. Certain vitamins and minerals, such as vitamin C, vitamin D, zinc, and selenium, play a crucial role in immune function. A well-nourished body is better equipped to fight off infections and diseases.

Individuality and Balance: It's important to recognize that nutrition needs can vary based on individual factors such as age, gender, activity level, and overall health. Moreover, achieving a balanced diet is about overall patterns and choices rather than focusing on individual foods. It's about moderation and incorporating a variety of nutrient-rich foods into our meals while allowing for occasional indulgences. Striving for balance and listening to our bodies' hunger and fullness cues is key.

In conclusion, nutrition plays a vital role in maintaining optimal health. A well-balanced and nutritious diet, comprising macronutrients, micronutrients, and adequate hydration, supports our physical, mental, and emotional well-being. By making informed food choices, we can prevent chronic diseases, manage weight, boost energy levels, support our immune system, and promote overall vitality. Embracing a healthy and balanced approach to nutrition is an investment in our long-term health and well-being.

The importance of sleep and stress management in overall wellness

The importance of sleep and stress management in overall wellness cannot be overstated. Both sleep and stress have a significant impact on our physical, mental, and emotional well-being. Let's explore why these aspects are crucial for maintaining a healthy and balanced life:

Sleep:

1. **Physical Restoration:** Sleep is a time of physical restoration and repair. During sleep, our bodies undergo processes such as tissue growth and repair, muscle recovery, and the release of hormones that regulate growth and appetite. Sufficient sleep allows our bodies to recover from daily activities and prepares us for optimal functioning the next day.

2. **Mental Clarity and Cognitive Function:** Quality sleep is essential for mental clarity, focus, and cognitive function. It enhances memory consolidation, information processing, problem-solving abilities, and creativity. Adequate sleep promotes optimal brain health and supports overall cognitive performance.

3. **Emotional Well-being:** Sleep plays a crucial role in regulating emotions and maintaining emotional well-being. Lack of sleep can contribute to mood disturbances, increased irritability, and heightened emotional reactivity. On the other hand, restful sleep improves emotional resilience and fosters a positive mood.

4. **Immune System Support:** Sleep is closely linked to immune function. During sleep, our immune system works to fight off infections, heal wounds, and support overall immune health. Chronic sleep deprivation can weaken the immune system, making us more susceptible to illnesses and infections.

5. **Hormonal Balance:** Sleep is intricately connected to hormonal balance. Insufficient sleep disrupts the production and regulation of hormones, including those involved in appetite control, metabolism, and stress response. This can contribute to weight gain, increased appetite, and imbalances in insulin and blood sugar levels.

Stress Management:

1. **Physical Health:** Chronic stress has detrimental effects on our physical health. Prolonged exposure to stress hormones, such as cortisol, can contribute to high blood pressure, cardiovascular diseases, weakened immune system, and digestive disorders. Managing stress is crucial for maintaining optimal physical health and reducing the risk of stress-related illnesses.

2. **Mental Well-being:** Unmanaged stress can significantly impact our mental health. It increases the risk of anxiety, depression, and other mood disorders. Effective stress management techniques, such as relaxation exercises, mindfulness, and engaging in activities we enjoy, can help reduce stress levels and promote emotional well-being.

3. **Cognitive Function:** Stress can impair cognitive function, including memory, attention, and decision-making abilities. Chronic stress can negatively affect our ability to concentrate, process information, and perform well in various tasks. By managing stress, we can optimize cognitive function and enhance overall productivity.

4. **Sleep Quality:** Stress and sleep are interconnected. Stress can interfere with sleep patterns, making it difficult to fall asleep or stay asleep. On the other hand, lack of quality sleep can increase stress levels. Implementing stress management strategies can help improve sleep quality and create a positive cycle of relaxation and rest.

5. **Relationships and Social Well-being:** Chronic stress can strain relationships and hinder social connections. Effective stress management techniques allow us to better communicate, handle conflicts, and maintain healthy relationships. Nurturing social connections and seeking support from loved ones can also be beneficial for managing stress.

In summary, prioritizing sleep and effective stress management are essential for overall wellness. Quality sleep allows for physical restoration, supports mental clarity, and promotes emotional well-being. Managing stress helps maintain physical and mental health, enhances cognitive function, and fosters positive relationships. By incorporating healthy sleep habits and stress management techniques into our lives, we can achieve a state of balance, resilience, and overall well-being.

Chapter 2: Building a Solid Fitness Routine

Embarking on a fitness journey is an empowering decision that can have transformative effects on our physical, mental, and emotional well-being. Building a solid fitness routine is the foundation upon which we can achieve our health and fitness goals, and ultimately, lead a more vibrant and fulfilling life. In this chapter, we will explore the key elements of creating a sustainable and effective fitness routine that caters to our individual needs and preferences.

The concept of a fitness routine extends beyond sporadic workouts or temporary bursts of motivation. It involves a systematic approach to incorporating physical activity into our daily lives and making it a lifelong commitment. By establishing a routine, we create structure, consistency, and accountability, which are essential for achieving long-term results and maintaining a healthy lifestyle.

This chapter will guide you through the process of building a solid fitness routine that encompasses various aspects, including goal setting, exercise selection, frequency, duration, and progression. We will explore the importance of incorporating different types of exercises to ensure a well-rounded and balanced approach to fitness. Additionally, we will discuss strategies for overcoming common obstacles and staying motivated on our fitness journey.

Understanding our unique goals and priorities is the first step in designing a fitness routine that aligns with our needs and aspirations. Whether our goals involve weight loss, strength gain, improved cardiovascular fitness, or overall well-being, a tailored fitness routine can help us reach those milestones.

Furthermore, we will delve into the significance of setting realistic and measurable goals that provide a sense of direction and purpose. By establishing clear objectives, we can track our progress, celebrate achievements, and adjust our routine as necessary.

In this chapter, we will also address the importance of considering individual factors such as fitness level, age, health condition, and time availability when designing a fitness routine. A personalized approach ensures that our routine is safe, sustainable, and enjoyable, reducing the risk of injuries and promoting long-term adherence.

Moreover, we will explore the concept of progressive overload, which involves gradually increasing the intensity, duration, or frequency of our workouts over time. This principle is crucial for continually challenging our bodies, promoting adaptations, and achieving ongoing improvements in fitness levels.

Lastly, we will discuss strategies for staying motivated and overcoming common obstacles that may hinder our fitness journey. We will explore techniques such as finding accountability partners, seeking professional guidance, varying our workouts, and celebrating small victories to maintain enthusiasm and commitment.

Building a solid fitness routine is not about perfection or adhering to strict rules. It is about creating a framework that allows us to engage in regular physical activity, enjoy the process, and continually strive for self-improvement. By incorporating the principles and strategies outlined in this chapter, we can lay the groundwork for a successful fitness journey that supports our overall health, well-being, and longevity. So, let's embark on this exciting adventure of creating a sustainable fitness routine that empowers us to become the best version of ourselves.

Assessing your current fitness level and setting realistic goals

Assessing your current fitness level and setting realistic goals is a crucial step in building a solid fitness routine. This process allows you to establish a baseline, understand your strengths and areas for improvement, and design a plan that is tailored to your individual needs and capabilities. By setting realistic goals, you can create a roadmap for your fitness journey and increase your chances of success. Let's explore this topic in detail:

Assessing Your Current Fitness Level:

- **Physical Fitness Components:** Assessing your current fitness level involves evaluating various physical fitness components, including cardiovascular endurance, muscular strength and endurance, flexibility, and body composition. These components provide a holistic view of your overall fitness and help identify areas that may require more attention.

- **Cardiovascular Endurance:** Assessing cardiovascular endurance involves measuring how efficiently your heart and lungs can deliver oxygen to your muscles during prolonged physical activity. Common assessments include timed runs or walks, cycling tests, or step tests.

- **Muscular Strength and Endurance:** This assessment focuses on evaluating the strength and endurance of your major muscle groups. It can involve exercises like push-ups, squats, or lifting weights to determine your maximum strength or the number of repetitions you can perform.

- **Flexibility:** Flexibility assessments measure your range of motion around various joints. These assessments may include stretches to evaluate the flexibility of major muscle groups, such as hamstring stretches or shoulder mobility tests.

- **Body Composition:** Assessing body composition helps determine the proportion of fat, muscle, and other tissues in your body. Methods such as skinfold calipers, bioelectrical impedance analysis, or DEXA scans can provide valuable insights into your body composition.

Functional Fitness Assessments:

In addition to the physical fitness components, functional fitness assessments evaluate your ability to perform daily tasks and movements efficiently. These assessments focus on activities such as balance, coordination, agility, and core stability. Functional fitness assessments can include exercises like balance tests, agility drills, or functional movement screenings.

Seeking Professional Guidance:

While self-assessment can provide valuable information, consulting with a fitness professional, such as a certified personal trainer or exercise physiologist, can offer more accurate and comprehensive assessments. Fitness professionals have the expertise to conduct specific tests, interpret the results, and provide tailored recommendations based on your goals and abilities.

Setting Realistic Goals:

SMART Goals: Setting goals that are Specific, Measurable, Achievable, Relevant, and Time-bound (SMART) is key to ensuring they are realistic and attainable. SMART goals provide clarity, motivation, and a clear timeline for achieving your desired outcomes.

Specific: Clearly define your goal. For example, instead of stating "I want to get fit," specify "I want to improve my cardiovascular endurance by running a 5K race."

Measurable: Establish measurable criteria to track your progress and success. For example, set a target time or distance for your 5K race, such as completing it in under 30 minutes.

Achievable: Ensure your goal is realistic and attainable within your current fitness level and circumstances. Consider factors such as time availability, physical capabilities, and other commitments.

Relevant: Align your goals with your overall aspirations, values, and priorities. Make sure they are meaningful and relevant to you personally.

Time-bound: Set a specific timeframe for achieving your goal. This provides a sense of urgency and helps you stay focused and motivated. For example, aim to complete your 5K race within three months.

Short-Term and Long-Term Goals:

It is beneficial to set both short-term and long-term goals. Short-term goals can be achievable within a few weeks or months and serve as stepping stones towards your long-term objectives. Long-term goals provide a broader vision and may span several months or years. Breaking down your goals into smaller milestones makes them more manageable and allows you to celebrate achievements along the way.

Consider Individual Factors:

When setting goals, consider your current fitness level, age, health condition, and lifestyle factors. Be honest with yourself about what you can realistically achieve given your circumstances. Setting goals that are too ambitious or unrealistic can lead to frustration, setbacks, and even injuries. It is essential to find the right balance between challenging yourself and setting attainable goals.

Adjusting Goals:

Remember that goals are not set in stone. As you progress on your fitness journey, it is natural to reassess and adjust your goals. You may find that you surpass your initial expectations or encounter obstacles that require modifications. Regularly evaluate your goals, monitor your progress, and make adjustments as needed to ensure they remain relevant and achievable.

In conclusion, assessing your current fitness level and setting realistic goals are fundamental steps in building a solid fitness routine. By evaluating your physical fitness components, functional abilities, and seeking professional guidance when needed, you gain valuable insights into your strengths and areas for improvement. Setting SMART goals that are specific, measurable, achievable, relevant, and time-bound provides a roadmap for your fitness journey and increases your chances of success. Consider individual factors and regularly reassess and adjust your goals to ensure they align with your capabilities and aspirations. By setting realistic goals, you set yourself up for a sustainable and fulfilling fitness journey that promotes overall health and well-being.

Designing a personalized workout plan

Designing a personalized workout plan is the key to achieving your fitness goals and maintaining a consistent exercise routine. A well-designed plan takes into account your individual needs, preferences, fitness level, and specific objectives. By tailoring your workouts to suit your unique circumstances, you can optimize your progress, prevent plateaus, and increase your motivation to stick with it. In this chapter, we will explore the essential components of a personalized workout plan and how to incorporate various types of exercises for maximum effectiveness.

Cardiovascular exercises and their benefits

Cardiovascular exercises, also known as aerobic exercises, are activities that increase your heart rate and breathing rate over an extended period. These exercises work your cardiovascular system, strengthening your heart and lungs, and improving overall endurance. Some common examples of cardiovascular exercises include running, swimming, cycling, dancing, and brisk walking.

The benefits of cardiovascular exercises are numerous. Firstly, they enhance cardiovascular health by improving the efficiency of your heart and lungs. Regular cardiovascular exercise can reduce the risk of heart disease, lower blood pressure, and improve cholesterol levels. Additionally, these exercises help in burning calories and promoting weight loss, making them an essential component of any fitness plan aimed at shedding excess pounds. Cardiovascular exercises also boost mood and mental well-being by releasing endorphins, reducing stress, and improving sleep quality. Incorporating regular cardio workouts into your personalized plan will not only improve your physical fitness but also contribute to your overall health and well-being.

Strength training and muscle development

Strength training exercises involve resistance or weight-bearing activities that target your muscles and build strength, power, and endurance. These exercises can be performed using free weights, weight machines, resistance bands, or your body weight. Strength training is crucial for preserving and building lean muscle mass, which plays a vital role in increasing metabolism, improving posture, and enhancing overall body composition.

One of the primary benefits of strength training is the development of stronger muscles and bones. It helps to prevent age-related muscle loss, maintain joint stability, and reduce the risk of osteoporosis. Strength training also enhances functional fitness, enabling you to perform daily tasks with ease and reducing the risk of injuries. Additionally, it provides a metabolic boost, as muscle tissue burns more calories at rest compared to fat tissue. This makes strength training an effective tool for weight management and long-term weight loss.

When designing your personalized workout plan, incorporate a variety of strength training exercises that target different muscle groups. Focus on compound exercises, such as squats, deadlifts, bench presses, and pull-ups, as they engage multiple muscles simultaneously. It is also important to gradually increase the intensity and resistance over time to continually challenge your muscles and promote progress.

Flexibility and mobility exercises

Flexibility exercises are designed to improve joint range of motion, muscle elasticity, and overall flexibility. These exercises include stretching, yoga, and other mobility drills. Incorporating flexibility exercises into your workout plan is essential for preventing injuries, maintaining proper posture, and enhancing athletic performance.

By regularly engaging in flexibility exercises, you can improve your joint mobility, which allows for a full range of motion during other exercises and activities. Stretching and mobility drills also help alleviate muscle stiffness and soreness, increase blood flow to muscles, and promote relaxation and stress reduction. Improved flexibility can enhance athletic performance by facilitating better movement mechanics, balance, and coordination.

When designing your workout plan, allocate dedicated time for flexibility exercises. Include dynamic stretches as part of your warm-up routine to prepare your muscles and joints for the workout ahead. Post-workout, incorporate static stretches to help cool down your body and promote muscle recovery. Consider attending yoga classes or using online resources to learn and practice different stretching techniques for maximum flexibility benefits.

Incorporating interval training for maximum results

Interval training involves alternating periods of high-intensity exercise with periods of low-intensity recovery or rest. This type of training is highly effective for boosting cardiovascular fitness, burning calories, and improving overall endurance. Interval training can be applied to various forms of cardiovascular exercises, such as running, cycling, swimming, or even jump rope.

The key benefit of interval training is its ability to increase the efficiency of your workouts in a shorter amount of time. By pushing your body to its maximum capacity during the high-intensity intervals, you stimulate cardiovascular improvements and metabolic adaptations. The short recovery periods allow for brief rest and prevent excessive fatigue, enabling you to sustain a higher overall intensity throughout the workout.

To incorporate interval training into your personalized workout plan, identify appropriate exercises and determine the duration and intensity of the intervals and recovery periods. Start with shorter intervals and gradually increase the intensity and duration as your fitness level improves. Interval training can be adapted to suit different fitness levels and preferences, making it a versatile and effective tool for achieving your goals.

In conclusion, designing a personalized workout plan involves carefully considering cardiovascular exercises, strength training, flexibility exercises, and the incorporation of interval training. By incorporating a variety of exercises into your plan, you can target different aspects of fitness, prevent boredom, and achieve optimal results. Remember to assess your current fitness level, set realistic goals, and progress gradually to avoid injury and maintain long-term adherence to your plan.

Chapter 3: Mastering Nutritional Balance

Mastering Nutritional Balance explores the crucial role of nutrition in achieving optimal health and fitness. While exercise is essential for physical fitness, nutrition plays an equally vital role in fueling the body, promoting recovery, and supporting overall well-being. This chapter delves into the fundamental principles of nutritional balance, providing valuable insights and practical guidelines to help you make informed choices about what you eat.

Understanding the relationship between nutrition and health is paramount. A well-balanced diet provides the necessary nutrients, vitamins, minerals, and energy to support bodily functions, maintain a healthy weight, and reduce the risk of chronic diseases. Nutrition not only affects our physical health but also influences our mental and emotional well-being, energy levels, cognitive function, and athletic performance.

In this chapter, we will explore various aspects of nutritional balance, including macronutrients (carbohydrates, proteins, and fats), micronutrients (vitamins and minerals), hydration, and mindful eating. We will examine how these components work together to optimize our health and support our fitness goals. By understanding the foundations of a nutritious diet and learning practical strategies for implementation, you will be empowered to make informed choices that align with your individual needs and objectives.

Additionally, we will address common myths and misconceptions surrounding nutrition, such as fad diets, quick fixes, and restrictive eating patterns. It's important to approach nutrition with a balanced and sustainable mindset, focusing on long-term habits rather than short-term trends. We will emphasize the importance of developing a healthy relationship with food, promoting intuitive eating, and finding joy in nourishing your body with wholesome, delicious meals.

Moreover, we will explore the significance of meal planning and preparation for maintaining consistency in your nutritional intake. By learning effective strategies for meal prepping, grocery shopping, and mindful eating, you can overcome common barriers to healthy eating, such as time constraints and unhealthy food temptations. We will provide practical tips and resources to help you establish sustainable habits that align with your lifestyle and goals.

Remember, nutrition is a journey of self-discovery and continuous learning. What works for one person may not work for another, as individual needs and preferences vary. By embracing the principles of nutritional balance and applying them in a way that suits your unique circumstances, you can fuel your body, support your fitness endeavors, and cultivate a lifelong foundation of health and well-being.

In the following chapters, we will delve deeper into the key aspects of nutritional balance, exploring macronutrients, micronutrients, hydration, and mindful eating. We will provide evidence-based recommendations, practical tips, and real-life examples to help you navigate the complex world of nutrition and develop a sustainable, nourishing approach to food. Remember, small changes can lead to significant results, and with the right knowledge and mindset, you can master the art of nutritional balance.

Understanding macronutrients (carbohydrates, proteins, and fats) and their functions

Macronutrients are essential components of our diet that provide the body with energy and play crucial roles in supporting overall health and well-being. The three primary macronutrients are carbohydrates, proteins, and fats. Understanding these macronutrients and their functions is key to achieving a well-balanced and nutritious diet. Let's explore each macronutrient in detail:

1. **Carbohydrates: Carbohydrates are the body's primary source of energy. They are broken down into glucose, which is used by the cells for fuel. Carbohydrates can be categorized into two types: simple and complex. Simple carbohydrates, found in fruits, honey, and refined sugars, are quickly digested and provide a rapid burst of energy. Complex carbohydrates, found in whole grains, legumes, and vegetables, are digested more slowly, providing sustained energy and a feeling of fullness.**

Carbohydrates serve several functions in the body:

- **Energy production:** As the body's preferred energy source, carbohydrates fuel various bodily functions, including physical activity and brain function.

- **Glycogen storage:** Excess glucose is stored in the muscles and liver as glycogen, which can be used later when energy demands increase.

- **Fiber:** Certain carbohydrates, particularly those found in whole grains, fruits, and vegetables, provide dietary fiber. Fiber aids in digestion, promotes feelings of fullness, and helps maintain healthy bowel movements.

2. **Proteins: Proteins are essential for growth, repair, and maintenance of body tissues. They are made up of amino acids, which are the building blocks of proteins. While the body can synthesize some amino acids, there are nine essential amino acids that must be obtained through the diet.**

Proteins serve several functions in the body:

- **Tissue repair and growth:** Proteins are involved in the repair and regeneration of tissues, including muscles, organs, skin, and hair.

- **Enzyme production:** Enzymes are proteins that catalyze various chemical reactions in the body, facilitating processes such as digestion and metabolism.

- **Hormone production:** Some hormones, such as insulin and growth hormone, are made up of protein structures and play important roles in regulating bodily functions.

- **Immune system support:** Antibodies, which are proteins, are vital components of the immune system and help defend against pathogens.

It's important to consume a variety of protein sources to ensure an adequate intake of all essential amino acids. Good sources of protein include lean meats, poultry, fish, eggs, dairy products, legumes, nuts, and seeds.

3. **Fats:** Fats, also known as lipids, are a concentrated source of energy and play essential roles in the body's functioning. They provide insulation and protection to organs, aid in the absorption of fat-soluble vitamins (A, D, E, and K), and serve as a source of essential fatty acids.

Fats can be divided into different categories:

- **Saturated fats:** Found in animal products such as meat and dairy, as well as some plant-based oils like coconut and palm oil. Consuming excessive amounts of saturated fats may increase the risk of heart disease and should be limited.

- **Unsaturated fats:** These can be further categorized into monounsaturated fats (found in olive oil, avocados, and nuts) and polyunsaturated fats (found in fatty fish, flaxseeds, and walnuts). Unsaturated fats, particularly omega-3 and omega-6 fatty acids, are important for brain function, reducing inflammation, and supporting heart health.

- **Trans-fats:** These fats are artificially produced through a process called hydrogenation and are commonly found in processed and fried foods. Trans-fats have been linked to an increased risk of heart disease and should be avoided as much as possible.

While fats are a concentrated source of calories, they are an important part of a balanced diet. Aim to include healthy fats in your diet while moderating your overall fat intake.

It's important to note that the optimal distribution of macronutrients in your diet may vary depending on individual needs, goals, and preferences. Consulting with a healthcare professional or registered dietitian can help determine the appropriate macronutrient ratios for your specific needs.

In summary, macronutrients are vital components of a well-balanced diet. Carbohydrates provide energy, proteins support tissue repair and growth, and fats play important roles in various bodily functions. By understanding the functions and sources of these macronutrients, you can make informed choices and create a nutritionally balanced diet that supports your health and fitness goals.

The significance of micronutrients (vitamins and minerals) in a healthy diet

Micronutrients, including vitamins and minerals, are essential components of a healthy diet. While they are required in smaller quantities compared to macronutrients, their role in supporting overall health and well-being cannot be overstated. Micronutrients are involved in numerous physiological processes in the body, ranging from immune function and energy production to cell growth and repair. Let's explore the significance of micronutrients in more detail:

Vitamins: Vitamins are organic compounds that are necessary for various biochemical reactions in the body. They are classified into two categories: water-soluble vitamins (B vitamins and vitamin C) and fat-soluble vitamins (vitamins A, D, E, and K).

Water-soluble vitamins are not stored in the body, so they need to be consumed regularly. They play vital roles in energy metabolism, cell division, and the functioning of the nervous system. B vitamins, such as thiamin, riboflavin, niacin, vitamin B6, vitamin B12, and folate, are involved in energy production and the synthesis of red blood cells. Vitamin C acts as an antioxidant, supporting immune function, collagen synthesis, and iron absorption.

Fat-soluble vitamins are stored in the body's fat tissues and the liver. They require dietary fats for absorption. Vitamin A is essential for vision, immune function, and the health of skin and mucous membranes. Vitamin D plays a crucial role in bone health, as it aids in the absorption of calcium and phosphorus. Vitamin E acts as an antioxidant, protecting cells from damage, while vitamin K is involved in blood clotting and bone metabolism.

Minerals: Minerals are inorganic substances that the body needs for various physiological functions. They are classified into two categories: major minerals (required in larger amounts) and trace minerals (required in smaller amounts).

Major minerals include calcium, phosphorus, magnesium, sodium, potassium, and chloride. These minerals are involved in maintaining electrolyte balance, regulating fluid balance, supporting muscle contraction, and building and maintaining strong bones.

Trace minerals, such as iron, zinc, copper, manganese, iodine, selenium, and chromium, are essential for several bodily functions. Iron is crucial for the formation of red blood cells and oxygen transport. Zinc is involved in immune function, wound healing, and DNA synthesis. Copper supports the formation of connective tissues and assists in iron metabolism. Manganese plays a role in bone formation and antioxidant defense. Iodine is necessary for thyroid hormone production, which regulates metabolism, growth, and development. Selenium acts as an antioxidant and is involved in thyroid hormone metabolism. Chromium plays a role in carbohydrate and lipid metabolism.

The significance of Micronutrients: Micronutrients play critical roles in maintaining optimal health and preventing nutrient deficiencies. They are involved in a wide range of functions, including:

- Energy production: Micronutrients are required as cofactors in enzymatic reactions involved in the breakdown of carbohydrates, proteins, and fats to produce energy.

- Immune function: Several vitamins and minerals, such as vitamins A, C, D, E, zinc, and selenium, support immune function, helping the body fight off infections and diseases.

- Cell growth and repair: Micronutrients are involved in DNA synthesis, cell division, and the production of new cells, supporting tissue growth, repair, and regeneration.

- Antioxidant defense: Many vitamins, such as vitamin C and vitamin E, and minerals, such as selenium and copper, act as antioxidants, protecting cells from oxidative damage caused by free radicals.

- Bone health: Micronutrients like calcium, phosphorus, magnesium, vitamin D, and vitamin K are crucial for maintaining strong bones and preventing conditions like osteoporosis.

- Nervous system function: B vitamins, particularly thiamin, riboflavin, niacin, vitamin B6, and vitamin B12, are essential for the proper functioning of the nervous system and the synthesis of neurotransmitters.

Obtaining Micronutrients: A well-balanced diet rich in fruits, vegetables, whole grains, lean proteins, and healthy fats is the best way to obtain a wide array of micronutrients. Different foods contain different micronutrients, so it's important to consume a variety of nutrient-dense foods to ensure an adequate intake.

In some cases, dietary supplementation may be necessary, especially for individuals with specific deficiencies or special dietary needs. However, it's important to note that supplements should not replace a balanced diet and should be taken under the guidance of a healthcare professional.

In conclusion, micronutrients, including vitamins and minerals, are essential for maintaining optimal health and well-being. They play critical roles in various bodily functions, supporting energy production, immune function, cell growth and repair, antioxidant defense, bone health, and nervous system function. By consuming a diverse range of nutrient-dense foods, you can ensure an adequate intake of micronutrients, supporting your overall health and vitality.

Creating a balanced meal plan

Creating a balanced meal plan is an effective way to ensure that you are meeting your nutritional needs and maintaining a healthy diet. A balanced meal plan involves incorporating a variety of foods from different food groups in appropriate portions to provide essential nutrients and support overall well-being. By following a balanced meal plan, you can optimize your energy levels, support your body's functions, and achieve your health and fitness goals. Let's explore the key components of creating a balanced meal plan:

1. Determine your calorie needs: Before creating a meal plan, it's important to determine your daily calorie needs based on factors such as age, gender, weight, activity level, and goals. Caloric requirements vary for each individual, so consulting with a registered dietitian or using online tools and calculators can help you estimate your calorie needs accurately.

2. Include macronutrients: A balanced meal plan should include appropriate amounts of macronutrients: carbohydrates, proteins, and fats.

   - Carbohydrates: Choose complex carbohydrates such as whole grains, legumes, fruits, and vegetables. These provide fiber, vitamins, and minerals while releasing energy slowly.

   - Proteins: Include lean sources of protein like poultry, fish, eggs, legumes, tofu, and dairy products. These provide essential amino acids for muscle repair, immune function, and overall health.

   - Fats: Incorporate healthy fats from sources such as avocados, nuts, seeds, olive oil, and fatty fish. These fats provide essential fatty acids and support various bodily functions.

3. Prioritize fruits and vegetables: Fruits and vegetables are packed with vitamins, minerals, antioxidants, and fiber. Aim to include a variety of colorful fruits and vegetables in your meals. They can be consumed fresh, frozen, or cooked and can be incorporated into main dishes, side dishes, salads, smoothies, or snacks.

4. Choose whole grains: Select whole grains over refined grains to benefit from their higher fiber content and greater nutrient density. Include options such as whole wheat bread, brown rice, quinoa, oats, and whole grain pasta.

5. Include lean sources of protein: Choose lean sources of protein to minimize saturated fat intake. Opt for skinless poultry, fish, lean cuts of meat, eggs, low-fat dairy products, legumes, and plant-based protein sources like tofu and tempeh.

6. Don't forget about healthy fats: Incorporate healthy fats into your meals to support heart health and provide satiety. Include sources such as avocados, nuts, seeds, olives, and oils like olive oil and avocado oil. However, remember that fats are calorie-dense, so portion control is important.

7. Incorporate dairy or dairy alternatives: If you consume dairy products, choose low-fat or fat-free options to limit saturated fat intake. If you're lactose intolerant or follow a vegan diet, opt for fortified plant-based milk alternatives like almond milk, soy milk, or oat milk.

8. Mindful portion control: While focusing on food choices is crucial, portion control is equally important. Be mindful of portion sizes to avoid overeating and to maintain a healthy weight. Use visual cues or measuring tools initially to develop a better understanding of appropriate portion sizes.

9. Plan and prep your meals: To stay consistent with your balanced meal plan, consider meal planning and prepping. Set aside time each week to plan your meals, create a grocery list, and prepare some components in advance. This can help you make healthier choices, save time, and reduce the likelihood of resorting to unhealthy options when you're busy or tired.

10. Stay hydrated: Don't forget the importance of hydration in a balanced meal plan. Water should be your primary beverage choice. Aim to drink adequate water throughout the day and limit the consumption of sugary drinks, sodas, and excessive caffeine.

Remember, a balanced meal plan is not a rigid prescription but rather a flexible framework that can be tailored to your individual preferences and dietary needs. It's essential to listen to your body, honor your hunger and fullness cues, and make adjustments as necessary. Consulting with a registered dietitian can provide personalized guidance and support in creating a balanced meal plan that aligns with your specific goals and needs.

In conclusion, a balanced meal plan is key to providing your body with essential nutrients, maintaining energy levels, and supporting overall health and well-being. By including a variety of foods from different food groups in appropriate portions, you can create a meal plan that meets your nutritional needs and helps you achieve your health and fitness goals. With consistency and mindful eating, a balanced meal plan can contribute to long-term success in maintaining a healthy lifestyle.

Strategies for portion control and mindful eating

Strategies for portion control and mindful eating are essential tools for maintaining a balanced and healthy diet. These practices help you develop a better understanding of your body's hunger and fullness cues, prevent overeating, and promote a more mindful relationship with food. By incorporating these strategies into your eating habits, you can achieve better portion control and make more conscious choices about what and how much you eat. Let's explore some effective strategies for portion control and mindful eating:

1. Use smaller plates and bowls: Opt for smaller-sized plates and bowls to visually create the perception of a fuller plate. This can help you feel satisfied with smaller portions, as the plate appears more filled.

2. Measure portions: Use measuring cups, spoons, and a kitchen scale to measure your food portions, especially when you are first starting to practice portion control. This

helps you become more aware of appropriate serving sizes and prevents overestimation.

3. Fill half your plate with vegetables: Prioritize vegetables as they are low in calories and high in fiber, providing a feeling of fullness. By filling half your plate with vegetables, you naturally reduce the space available for higher-calorie foods.

4. Slow down and savor each bite: Eating mindfully involves slowing down the pace of your meals and fully savoring each bite. Take the time to chew your food thoroughly, appreciate the flavors and textures, and pay attention to your body's signals of hunger and fullness.

5. Listen to your body's cues: Tune in to your body's hunger and fullness cues to guide your eating habits. Eat when you are genuinely hungry and stop eating when you feel comfortably full. Avoid eating out of boredom, stress, or emotions.

6. Practice portioned snacking: If you enjoy snacking, pre-portion your snacks into small containers or bags to avoid mindlessly eating large quantities. This helps you keep track of your intake and prevents overindulgence.

7. Be aware of emotional eating: Recognize the difference between physical hunger and emotional hunger. Emotional eating involves eating to cope with emotions rather than actual hunger. Find alternative strategies to deal with emotions, such as engaging in hobbies, practicing mindfulness, or seeking support from loved ones.

8. Minimize distractions during meals: Avoid eating in front of screens or engaging in other distracting activities. Instead, create a calm and pleasant eating environment that allows you to focus on your food, appreciate the flavors, and recognize your body's satiety signals.

9. Practice mindful food choices: When deciding what to eat, consider the nutritional value of foods and how they make you feel. Choose whole, unprocessed foods that nourish your body and provide sustained energy. Be mindful of portion sizes when indulging in higher-calorie foods.

10. Keep a food journal: Keeping a food journal can increase your awareness of portion sizes and eating patterns. Documenting what and how much you eat can help you identify areas where portion control can be improved and provide insights into emotional or mindless eating triggers.

11. Plan and prepare meals in advance: By planning and preparing your meals ahead of time, you have better control over portion sizes and can make healthier choices. It reduces reliance on convenience foods, which tend to have larger portion sizes and less nutritional value.

12. Practice the 80/20 rule: Allow flexibility in your eating habits by adopting the 80/20 rule. Strive to make healthy choices about 80% of the time while leaving room for indulgences and treats the remaining 20% of the time. This approach promotes balance and prevents feelings of deprivation.

13. Seek support: Changing eating habits can be challenging, and it can be helpful to seek support from friends, family, or a registered dietitian. Having someone to share your journey with, provide encouragement, and hold you accountable can increase your chances of success.

Remember, portion control and mindful eating are lifelong practices that require patience and consistency. It's essential to be kind to yourself and embrace progress rather than perfection. Over time, these strategies will become second nature, and you'll develop a healthier relationship with food, enjoying meals with awareness and satisfaction.

Healthy cooking techniques and recipe ideas

Healthy cooking techniques and recipe ideas are essential for creating nutritious and delicious meals. By choosing the right cooking methods and incorporating wholesome ingredients, you can enhance the nutritional value of your meals while still enjoying a wide variety of flavors. Let's explore some healthy cooking techniques and recipe ideas that can inspire you to create balanced and tasty dishes:

Steaming: Steaming is a gentle cooking method that helps retain the natural flavors, colors, and nutrients of foods. It involves using steam to cook ingredients without submerging them in water. Steamed vegetables, fish, and dumplings are popular examples of steamed dishes.

Recipe idea: Steamed broccoli and salmon with a squeeze of lemon juice and a sprinkle of herbs make for a simple and nutritious meal.

Grilling: Grilling adds a smoky flavor to foods without the need for excess oil. It allows the fat to drip away from the food, making it a healthier cooking option. Grilled chicken, vegetables, and fruits are popular choices.

Recipe idea: Marinate chicken breasts in a mixture of olive oil, lemon juice, garlic, and herbs, then grill them until cooked through. Serve with grilled vegetables for a flavorful and nutritious meal.

Stir-frying: Stir-frying involves quickly cooking small, bite-sized pieces of food in a hot pan or wok with minimal oil. It helps retain the texture and color of vegetables while cooking them quickly, preserving their nutrients.

Recipe idea: Stir-fry a mix of colorful vegetables like bell peppers, broccoli, carrots, and snow peas with lean protein (chicken, tofu, or shrimp) and a light sauce made from low-sodium soy sauce, garlic, and ginger.

Baking or roasting: Baking or roasting uses dry heat to cook food, resulting in a crispy exterior and tender interior. It requires little to no added oil, making it a healthier alternative to frying.

Poaching: Poaching involves cooking food in a liquid, such as water or broth, at a low temperature. It is a gentle method that helps retain the moisture and tenderness of proteins without adding excess fat.

Recipe idea: Poach a piece of white fish, such as cod or tilapia, in a flavorful broth with herbs, lemon slices, and a touch of salt. Serve it with steamed vegetables and quinoa for a light and healthy meal.

Using herbs and spices: Experimenting with herbs and spices is a great way to add flavor to your dishes without relying on excessive salt, sugar, or unhealthy sauces. They can transform a simple meal into a flavorful culinary experience.

Recipe idea: Season grilled chicken with a mix of herbs like rosemary, thyme, and oregano, along with a dash of paprika and black pepper, for a tasty and aromatic dish.

Incorporating whole grains: Replace refined grains with whole grains in your recipes to increase fiber content and overall nutritional value. Whole grains like brown rice, quinoa, barley, and whole wheat pasta provide more nutrients and promote satiety.

Recipe idea: Prepare a colorful salad with cooked quinoa, mixed greens, cherry tomatoes, cucumbers, avocado, and a light vinaigrette for a nutritious and satisfying meal.

Experimenting with plant-based proteins: Explore the world of plant-based proteins such as legumes, tofu, tempeh, and seitan. These options are rich in fiber and nutrients while being lower in saturated fat compared to animal proteins.

Recipe idea: Make a hearty vegetarian chili using kidney beans, black beans, and diced vegetables like bell peppers, onions, and tomatoes. Add spices like cumin and chili powder for extra flavor.

Mindful meal planning: Plan your meals in advance to ensure a well-rounded and balanced diet. This allows you to make healthier choices and reduces the reliance on processed or convenience foods.

Recipe idea: Prepare a weekly meal plan that includes a variety of recipes from different food groups, such as roasted chicken with vegetables, lentil soup, fish tacos with slaw, and a quinoa salad. This way, you can enjoy a diverse range of nutrients throughout the week.

Modifying recipes: Don't be afraid to modify existing recipes to make them healthier. Swap ingredients for healthier alternatives, reduce added sugars, or adjust portion sizes to meet your dietary needs.

Remember, healthy cooking is not about sacrificing taste but rather finding creative ways to enhance flavors while nourishing your body. By incorporating these cooking techniques and recipe ideas into your culinary repertoire, you can create nutritious and satisfying meals that support your overall health and well-being.

Chapter 4: Mind-Body Connection: Managing Stress and Emotions

In today's fast-paced and demanding world, managing stress and emotions is crucial for maintaining overall well-being. The mind-body connection plays a significant role in our health, and understanding how our thoughts, emotions, and physical state are interconnected can empower us to effectively manage stress, improve our mental health, and enhance our overall quality of life. Chapter 4 delves into the intricate relationship between the mind and body, providing valuable insights and practical strategies for managing stress and emotions.

In this chapter, we will explore various techniques and approaches that promote a healthy mind-body connection, allowing you to navigate life's challenges with resilience and emotional balance. By developing self-awareness, cultivating mindfulness, and implementing proven stress management strategies, you can enhance your ability to respond to stressors, regulate emotions, and create a more harmonious and fulfilling life.

Stress has become a prevalent aspect of modern life, affecting individuals of all ages and backgrounds. While stress itself is a natural response to demanding situations, prolonged and unmanaged stress can have detrimental effects on our physical and mental health. Chronic stress has been linked to conditions such as cardiovascular disease, weakened immune function, anxiety, and depression. Recognizing the impact of stress on our well-being underscores the importance of effectively managing it.

Emotions also play a vital role in our overall health and well-being. They influence our thoughts, behaviors, and physiological responses. By learning to understand and regulate our emotions, we can cultivate emotional intelligence, build resilience, and improve our relationships with ourselves and others.

The mind-body connection acknowledges that our mental and emotional states can influence our physical health, and vice versa. For instance, chronic stress can manifest in physical symptoms such as headaches, muscle tension, and digestive problems. Conversely, physical well-being, through practices like exercise and nutrition, can positively impact our mental and emotional states.

Throughout this chapter, we will explore a range of strategies for managing stress and emotions, including mindfulness practices, relaxation techniques, cognitive-behavioral approaches, and self-care strategies. These tools empower you to develop a deeper understanding of yourself, manage stressors effectively, and cultivate emotional well-being.

By embracing the mind-body connection and implementing these strategies into your daily life, you can create a more balanced, resilient, and fulfilling existence. Join us as we embark on this transformative journey of managing stress and emotions, and unlock the power of the mind-body connection to enhance your overall well-being.

Exploring the mind-body connection and its impact on health

The mind-body connection refers to the intricate relationship between our mental and emotional states and our physical health. It recognizes that our thoughts, emotions, beliefs, and attitudes can influence our physical well-being, and vice versa. Research has shown that the mind and body are interconnected systems that constantly communicate and interact with each other.

One way in which the mind-body connection impacts our health is through the influence of stress. When we experience stress, whether it's due to work pressures, relationship challenges, or other life circumstances, our bodies respond by activating the stress response system. This triggers the release of stress hormones like cortisol and adrenaline, preparing us for a fight-or-flight response. While this response can be helpful in acute situations, chronic or prolonged stress can have detrimental effects on our health.

Chronic stress can lead to a wide range of physical and mental health problems. It has been associated with an increased risk of conditions such as cardiovascular disease, high blood pressure, obesity, diabetes, gastrointestinal issues, and weakened immune function. Stress can also exacerbate existing health conditions and contribute to mental health disorders such as anxiety and depression.

The impact of the mind-body connection on health goes beyond stress. Our thoughts, beliefs, and attitudes can influence our behaviors and lifestyle choices, which in turn impact our physical well-being. For example, negative thought patterns and self-limiting beliefs can undermine our motivation to exercise, eat healthily, and engage in self-care activities. On the other hand, positive thoughts and a healthy mindset can promote behaviors that support overall health and well-being.

Conversely, our physical health can also influence our mental and emotional states. Engaging in regular physical activity has been shown to have numerous benefits for mental health, including reducing symptoms of depression and anxiety, improving mood, boosting self-esteem, and promoting better sleep. Exercise stimulates the release of endorphins, which are natural mood-boosting chemicals in the brain. Additionally, taking care of our physical health through proper nutrition, adequate sleep, and other self-care practices can positively impact our mental and emotional well-being.

Mind-body practices such as mindfulness meditation, yoga, tai chi, and deep breathing exercises are powerful tools for enhancing the mind-body connection and promoting overall health. These practices help cultivate awareness of our thoughts, emotions, and bodily sensations, allowing us to respond to stressors in a more balanced and constructive way. By incorporating these practices into our daily lives, we can reduce stress, improve emotional regulation, and enhance our overall well-being.

Exploring the mind-body connection and understanding its impact on health is essential for developing a holistic approach to wellness. By recognizing the interplay between our thoughts, emotions, and physical health, we can take proactive steps to optimize our well-being. This may include adopting stress management techniques, engaging in regular physical activity, practicing mindfulness, cultivating positive thoughts and beliefs, and seeking support when needed.

By embracing the mind-body connection, we can empower ourselves to make choices that support our overall health and well-being. It is a journey of self-discovery and self-care, where we learn to nurture and nourish both our minds and bodies. When we recognize and honor the profound connection between our mental and physical states, we open the door to a more integrated and vibrant existence.

Techniques for stress management and relaxation

Stress management and relaxation techniques are valuable tools for promoting mental and physical well-being in today's fast-paced world. These techniques help to reduce the negative effects of stress, improve overall resilience, and restore a sense of calm and balance. There are numerous effective techniques that can be incorporated into a stress-reducing routine. Let's explore some of these techniques:

Deep Breathing: Deep breathing exercises are simple yet powerful tools for relaxation. By focusing on slow, deep breaths, you activate the body's relaxation response, which helps reduce stress and promote a sense of calm. Practice diaphragmatic breathing by inhaling deeply through your nose, filling your belly with air, and exhaling slowly through your mouth.

Progressive Muscle Relaxation (PMR): PMR involves systematically tensing and relaxing different muscle groups in the body. By doing so, you can release tension and promote physical and mental relaxation. Start by tensing a muscle group, such as your shoulders, for a few seconds, then release and let the tension melt away. Move through different muscle groups, from head to toe, for a complete relaxation experience.

Guided Imagery: Guided imagery involves using your imagination to create a relaxing and peaceful mental image. You can listen to guided imagery recordings or create your own visualization. Close your eyes, imagine yourself in a serene setting, and engage all your senses to experience the calmness and tranquility of that place.

Mindfulness Meditation: Mindfulness meditation involves bringing your attention to the present moment, without judgment. By focusing on your breath, sensations in the body, or the sounds around you, you cultivate a state of mindfulness that promotes relaxation and reduces stress. Start with short meditation sessions and gradually increase the duration as you become more comfortable with the practice.

Journaling: Writing down your thoughts and feelings can be a cathartic and stress-reducing activity. Set aside a few minutes each day to journal about your experiences, emotions, and any stressors you may be facing. This process can help you gain clarity, process your emotions, and reduce stress by expressing yourself on paper.

Engaging in Hobbies: Participating in activities that bring you joy and relaxation is an excellent way to manage stress. Engage in hobbies such as painting, gardening, playing a musical instrument, or any activity that allows you to focus on the present moment and provides a sense of fulfillment.

Social Support: Connecting with loved ones and seeking support from a strong support network is crucial for managing stress. Share your thoughts and feelings with trusted friends or family members, or consider joining support groups where you can find understanding and empathy.

Physical Activity: Engaging in regular physical activity is not only beneficial for physical health but also for stress reduction. Exercise releases endorphins, which are natural mood-boosting chemicals in the brain. Find an activity that you enjoy, whether it's walking, jogging, dancing, or swimming, and make it a regular part of your routine.

Time Management: Effective time management can significantly reduce stress levels. Prioritize your tasks, set realistic goals, and break them down into smaller, manageable steps. Creating a structured and organized schedule can help reduce feelings of overwhelm and increase productivity.

Remember, different techniques work for different individuals, so it's important to find what resonates with you and incorporate it into your daily routine. Experiment with various stress management and relaxation techniques to discover which ones bring you the most peace and tranquility. By incorporating these practices into your life, you can effectively manage stress, enhance well-being, and promote a healthier and more balanced lifestyle.

The power of meditation and mindfulness practices

The power of meditation and mindfulness practices cannot be overstated when it comes to promoting overall well-being and managing stress. These ancient practices have been embraced by people across cultures and have gained significant recognition in the modern world for their profound benefits on mental, emotional, and physical health.

Meditation is a practice that involves training the mind to focus and redirect thoughts. It often involves finding a quiet and comfortable space, assuming a specific posture, and engaging in techniques that cultivate a sense of calm and heightened awareness. Mindfulness, on the other hand, is the practice of intentionally paying attention to the present moment without judgment. It involves fully engaging in the here and now, being aware of thoughts, emotions, bodily sensations, and the surrounding environment.

One of the key benefits of meditation and mindfulness practices is their ability to reduce stress and promote relaxation. By focusing the mind and redirecting attention to the present moment, meditation and mindfulness help break the cycle of negative thoughts, worries, and anxieties that contribute to stress. They provide a mental and emotional reset, allowing individuals to cultivate a sense of inner peace, clarity, and calmness. Regular meditation practice has been shown to lower levels of stress hormones, such as cortisol, and promote a more balanced and resilient stress response.

Furthermore, meditation and mindfulness practices enhance self-awareness and emotional regulation. They create a space for individuals to observe their thoughts, feelings, and bodily sensations without judgment or attachment. Through this awareness, individuals can develop a deeper understanding of their emotions, patterns of thinking, and reactions. This self-awareness allows for more intentional and skillful responses to stressors and challenges, reducing impulsive reactions and fostering emotional balance.

Research has also demonstrated the positive impact of meditation and mindfulness on mental health. Regular practice has been shown to reduce symptoms of anxiety and depression, increase feelings of happiness and well-being, and improve overall psychological functioning. By developing a non-judgmental and accepting attitude toward their thoughts and emotions, individuals can cultivate a more compassionate and gentle relationship with themselves, promoting a healthier mindset and improved mental well-being.

Moreover, meditation and mindfulness practices have physical health benefits. They have been associated with reduced blood pressure, improved immune function, better sleep quality, and enhanced pain management. By inducing a state of deep relaxation and reducing the physiological effects of stress, these practices support overall physical health and well-being.

Incorporating meditation and mindfulness into daily life can be transformative. It is important to note that these practices require consistency and commitment to experience their full benefits. Starting with short sessions and gradually increasing duration can help build a sustainable practice. There are various forms of meditation and mindfulness techniques to explore, including focused attention meditation, loving-kindness meditation, body scan meditation, and mindful walking, among others. Finding a practice that resonates with you and fits into your lifestyle is key.

To support a meditation and mindfulness practice, creating a dedicated space for practice, establishing a regular routine, and seeking guidance from experienced teachers or utilizing meditation apps can be helpful. Engaging in group meditation or mindfulness sessions can also provide a sense of community and support.

In conclusion, the power of meditation and mindfulness practices lies in their ability to cultivate a deep sense of presence, awareness, and inner peace. By incorporating these practices into our lives, we can reduce stress, enhance self-awareness and emotional regulation, improve mental health, and promote physical well-being. The transformative effects of meditation and mindfulness extend far beyond the moments of practice, influencing our overall perception, mindset, and relationship with ourselves and the world around us.

Emotional well-being and cultivating positive relationships

Emotional well-being and cultivating positive relationships are fundamental aspects of a fulfilling and balanced life. Our emotions play a significant role in shaping our thoughts, behaviors, and overall sense of happiness and satisfaction. Likewise, the quality of our relationships profoundly impacts our emotional well-being and contributes to our overall sense of belonging and connectedness.

Emotional well-being refers to our ability to understand, manage, and express our emotions in a healthy and constructive manner. It involves developing emotional intelligence, which encompasses self-awareness, self-regulation, empathy, and effective communication skills. Cultivating emotional well-being allows us to navigate life's ups and downs with resilience, build healthier relationships, and experience a greater sense of fulfillment.

One essential aspect of emotional well-being is developing self-awareness. Self-awareness involves understanding our own emotions, needs, and values. It requires taking time for self-reflection and introspection to explore our thoughts, beliefs, and patterns of behavior. By developing self-awareness, we gain insight into our emotions, triggers, and how they influence our thoughts and actions. This self-awareness enables us to make conscious choices and respond to situations in a way that aligns with our values and supports our emotional well-being.

Another important aspect of emotional well-being is self-regulation. Self-regulation involves the ability to manage our emotions effectively and respond to situations in a balanced and constructive manner. It entails recognizing and acknowledging our emotions without being overwhelmed by them. Through self-regulation, we can choose how to express our emotions in a way that is appropriate and considerate of others. Developing self-regulation skills allows us to maintain emotional balance, cope with stress, and navigate conflicts and challenges more effectively.

Empathy is a crucial component of emotional well-being and positive relationships. Empathy involves the ability to understand and share the emotions of others, putting ourselves in their shoes and offering support and understanding. By cultivating empathy, we build stronger connections with others, foster trust and mutual respect, and contribute to a more compassionate and harmonious social environment. Practicing empathy also enhances our own emotional well-being by fostering a sense of connection, empathy, and belonging.

Effective communication is a vital skill for cultivating positive relationships and emotional well-being. Good communication involves not only expressing our thoughts and feelings clearly but also actively listening and understanding others. It requires being attentive, validating the emotions of others, and responding with empathy and respect. By improving our communication skills, we can foster healthier relationships, resolve conflicts constructively, and create an environment where open and honest communication is valued.

Cultivating positive relationships is an essential part of emotional well-being. Healthy relationships provide support, love, and a sense of belonging. They contribute to our overall happiness and well-being by offering opportunities for connection, growth, and shared experiences. Building positive relationships involves investing time and effort in nurturing and maintaining them. It requires active listening, showing appreciation, being present, and practicing forgiveness and understanding.

To cultivate positive relationships, it is important to surround ourselves with people who uplift and inspire us, share similar values, and support our emotional well-being. Building a network of supportive relationships involves being proactive in seeking out social connections, participating in activities or communities that align with our interests, and being open to forming new friendships. It is also essential to invest in existing relationships by making time for quality interactions, engaging in meaningful conversations, and showing genuine care and empathy.

In conclusion, emotional well-being and cultivating positive relationships are vital components of a fulfilling and balanced life. By developing emotional intelligence, including self-awareness, self-regulation, empathy, and effective communication skills, we can enhance our emotional well-being and create healthier and more meaningful relationships. Nurturing positive relationships and investing in social connections provide a sense of belonging, support, and happiness, contributing to a more vibrant and satisfying life.

Chapter 5: Integrating Physical Activity into Everyday Life

In today's sedentary lifestyle, where technology and convenience have made physical activity optional rather than essential, it has become increasingly important to find ways to integrate movement and exercise into our daily routines. Chapter 5 focuses on the significance of incorporating physical activity into everyday life and explores strategies to make it a natural and enjoyable part of our routines.

Regular physical activity is crucial for maintaining optimal health and well-being. It not only helps in managing weight and preventing chronic diseases but also enhances mood, boosts energy levels, improves sleep quality, and promotes overall longevity. However, many people struggle to find the time and motivation to engage in dedicated exercise sessions.

The key to successfully integrating physical activity into everyday life lies in adopting a more active lifestyle rather than relying solely on structured workouts. This chapter will provide practical tips, techniques, and insights to help individuals embrace movement as a natural part of their daily routines, whether at work, home, or during leisure time.

By making physical activity a habitual and enjoyable part of our lives, we can overcome the barriers that often hinder consistent exercise. Whether it's finding creative ways to incorporate movement into our workdays, utilizing active transportation, or discovering enjoyable recreational activities, this chapter aims to inspire and empower readers to lead more active lives.

Through a combination of small, intentional changes and mindset shifts, individuals can transform their daily routines to include more movement and reap the benefits of an active lifestyle. From simple strategies like taking the stairs instead of the elevator, incorporating active breaks throughout the day, and engaging in active hobbies or sports, to finding support and accountability through social connections, this chapter will provide a comprehensive guide to integrating physical activity into everyday life.

By recognizing the value of movement in improving physical and mental well-being, individuals can break free from sedentary habits and discover the joy and fulfillment that comes from an active lifestyle. Through the practical advice and insights shared in this chapter, readers will gain the tools and knowledge needed to make physical activity a sustainable and enjoyable part of their everyday lives.

By embracing the philosophy of "movement as medicine," readers will be able to experience the positive impacts of increased activity on their overall health, productivity, and quality of life. From the moment they wake up to the time they go to bed, readers will be inspired to find creative ways to incorporate physical activity and movement into their daily routines, transforming their lives and nurturing a lifelong commitment to their well-being.

Incorporating exercise into a busy schedule

Incorporating exercise into a busy schedule can be a challenge, but it is not impossible. With some planning, creativity, and a commitment to prioritize your health, you can find ways to fit physical activity into even the busiest of days. This section explores various strategies and practical tips to help you integrate exercise seamlessly into your hectic schedule.

One of the first steps in incorporating exercise into a busy schedule is to make it a non-negotiable priority. Just as you allocate time for important work meetings or personal commitments, carve out dedicated time for exercise. Treat it as an essential appointment with yourself that cannot be canceled or rescheduled easily. By establishing this mindset, you will be more likely to follow through and make exercise a consistent part of your routine.

Efficiency is key when time is limited. Look for opportunities to incorporate short bursts of activity throughout your day. High-intensity interval training (HIIT) workouts are a great option as they can be completed in a short amount of time while still providing significant benefits. Consider setting aside 15-30 minutes during your lunch break or in the morning to engage in a quick HIIT session that gets your heart rate up and works your major muscle groups. These short bursts of intense exercise can be just as effective as longer workouts.

Another effective strategy is to maximize your daily activities by making them more active. For instance, if you commute to work, consider walking or biking instead of driving. If your workplace is too far, try parking your car farther away from the office and walk the remaining distance. Take the stairs instead of the elevator, and incorporate walking meetings or breaks into your workday. These small changes can add up and contribute to your overall physical activity level.

Utilize technology and online resources to your advantage. There are numerous fitness apps and websites that offer quick and effective workouts that can be done anywhere, anytime. From bodyweight exercises to yoga or Pilates routines, you can find a variety of options that suit your preferences and time constraints. By having access to guided workouts on your phone or computer, you can squeeze in a workout whenever you have a few spare minutes.

Consider incorporating exercise into your daily routine by multitasking. For example, you can listen to a podcast or audiobook while going for a brisk walk or run. If you enjoy watching TV shows or movies, use that time to engage in a workout. You can perform bodyweight exercises, use resistance bands, or even use a treadmill or stationary bike while enjoying your favorite entertainment. This way, you are maximizing your time and making exercise an enjoyable part of your leisure activities.

Lastly, seek support and accountability. Find a workout buddy or join a fitness group or class that aligns with your schedule. When you have a commitment to meet someone for a workout, you are more likely to follow through. Additionally, accountability partners can provide motivation, encouragement, and help you stay on track with your fitness goals.

Incorporating exercise into a busy schedule requires intention, planning, and flexibility. It may involve making sacrifices and rearranging priorities, but the long-term benefits to your physical and mental well-being make it worthwhile. By utilizing time-efficient workouts, maximizing daily activities, utilizing technology, multitasking, and seeking support, you can successfully integrate exercise into your busy schedule and enjoy the numerous health benefits that come with it. Remember, small steps and consistent effort lead to significant progress over time.

Active commuting and workplace fitness strategies

Active commuting and workplace fitness strategies are effective ways to incorporate physical activity into your daily routine, even when you have a busy schedule. This section explores the benefits of active commuting and provides practical tips for staying active at the workplace.

Active commuting refers to using physical activity as a means of transportation to and from work. Instead of relying solely on cars or public transportation, you can choose more active alternatives such as walking, cycling, or even running. Active commuting offers numerous benefits, including increased physical activity, reduced environmental impact, improved cardiovascular health, and reduced stress levels.

Walking or cycling to work allows you to incorporate exercise seamlessly into your daily routine. If the distance is manageable, consider walking or cycling the entire way. Alternatively, you can combine active commuting with public transportation by walking or cycling to a bus or train station and then continuing your journey from there. Not only does active commuting provide an opportunity to engage in physical activity, but it also helps you start your day with increased energy and a clear mind.

To make active commuting more convenient, consider planning your route in advance. Identify the safest and most suitable path, taking into account factors such as traffic, bike lanes, or pedestrian-friendly routes. Allow yourself some extra time to account for the physical activity involved in your commute. This way, you can enjoy a leisurely walk or bike ride without feeling rushed or stressed.

At the workplace, it's important to find ways to stay active throughout the day, especially if you have a sedentary job. Here are some workplace fitness strategies to consider:

1. **Take active breaks:** Instead of sitting for long periods, schedule regular breaks to move and stretch. Set reminders to stand up, walk around, or perform simple exercises like squats, lunges, or desk stretches. These short bursts of activity can help combat the negative effects of prolonged sitting.

2. **Walk or cycle during lunch:** Use your lunch break to engage in physical activity. Take a brisk walk or cycle outdoors if possible. If you have access to a gym or fitness facility nearby, consider using that time for a quick workout or fitness class.

3. **Use stairs instead of elevators:** Whenever possible, opt for the stairs instead of elevators or escalators. Climbing stairs is a great way to increase your heart rate, burn calories, and strengthen your leg muscles.

4. **Stand or use a standing desk:** If your workplace allows it, consider using a standing desk or a sit-stand workstation. Standing for periods throughout the day can help improve posture, increase calorie expenditure, and reduce the risk of certain health issues associated with prolonged sitting.

5. **Organize active group activities:** Encourage your colleagues to participate in group fitness activities or challenges. This could include lunchtime walks, office yoga or stretching sessions, or friendly competitions like step challenges or fitness classes. Engaging in activities as a group can create a supportive and motivating environment.

6. **Incorporate movement into meetings:** Instead of conducting all meetings sitting down, consider incorporating movement into some of them. Walking meetings or standing meetings can help promote creativity, engagement, and productivity, while also providing an opportunity to stay active.

Remember, consistency is key when it comes to incorporating physical activity into your daily routine. By making active commuting and workplace fitness strategies a regular part of your life, you can enjoy the benefits of increased physical activity, improved health, and enhanced well-being, even amidst a busy schedule.

Making fitness a family affair

Making fitness a family affair is a wonderful way to prioritize health and spend quality time together. When you involve your family in physical activities, you not only promote a healthy lifestyle but also create lasting memories and strengthen your relationships. This section explores the benefits of making fitness a family affair and provides practical tips for incorporating physical activities into your family routine.

1. **Promotes bonding:** Engaging in physical activities as a family allows you to bond and connect on a deeper level. Whether it's going for a hike, playing a game of soccer, or taking a family bike ride, these shared experiences create opportunities for meaningful conversations and laughter.

2. **Sets a positive example:** Children often learn by observing their parents' behavior. When they see you prioritize fitness and enjoy being active, they are more likely to develop healthy habits themselves. By making fitness a family value, you instill a lifelong commitment to health and well-being in your children.

3. **Provides quality time:** In today's busy world, finding quality time with your family can be a challenge. Incorporating physical activities into your routine allows you to spend meaningful time together, away from distractions like screens and technology. It creates an environment where you can engage with one another and enjoy each other's company.

4. **Builds healthy habits:** Regular physical activity is essential for children's physical and mental development. By engaging in fitness activities as a family, you establish a routine that promotes healthy habits and an active lifestyle. These habits can contribute to lifelong well-being and reduce the risk of chronic diseases later in life.

5. **Increases motivation and accountability:** Exercising as a family provides built-in motivation and accountability. When you have a workout buddy or a team cheering you on, it becomes easier to stay motivated and committed to your fitness goals. Encouraging and supporting each other creates a positive and supportive environment for everyone involved.

Now let's explore some practical tips for making fitness a family affair:

a) **Plan outdoor adventures:** Take advantage of nature by planning family hikes, nature walks, or bike rides. Explore local parks, trails, or nearby natural attractions. Encourage your children to appreciate the beauty of the outdoors while staying active.

b) **Engage in team sports:** Sign up for family-friendly team sports like soccer, basketball, or volleyball. Participating in organized leagues or friendly neighborhood games can be a fun way to stay active and encourage friendly competition.

c) **Play active games:** Organize family game nights that involve physical activities. Consider games like tag, hide-and-seek, relay races, or even backyard obstacle courses. These games provide opportunities for laughter, teamwork, and physical exertion.

d) **Take family walks or runs:** Schedule regular walks or runs as a family. Choose a scenic route or explore different neighborhoods together. You can also participate in local charity walks or fun runs, which not only promote fitness but also support meaningful causes.

e) **Try new activities together:** Explore a variety of physical activities as a family. Consider activities like swimming, dancing, martial arts, or yoga. Trying new activities together allows everyone to discover their interests and strengths while promoting overall fitness.

f) **Turn chores into fitness opportunities:** Involve your family in household chores that require physical activity. Gardening, cleaning, or rearranging furniture can be transformed into fun and active tasks that engage everyone in movement.

g) **Incorporate active vacations:** When planning family vacations, opt for destinations that offer opportunities for physical activities. Choose locations near beaches, mountains, or national parks that allow for hiking, swimming, or other outdoor adventures.

Remember, the key to making fitness a family affair is to prioritize fun and enjoyment. Focus on activities that everyone in the family can participate in and adjust the intensity according to individual fitness levels. By making fitness a shared experience, you create a positive and supportive environment that nurtures both physical and emotional well-being within your family.

Embracing outdoor activities and nature's benefits

Embracing outdoor activities and enjoying the benefits of nature is not only a great way to stay active but also to enhance your overall well-being. Spending time outdoors provides a refreshing change of scenery, fresh air, and the opportunity to connect with nature. This section explores the benefits of outdoor activities and how they contribute to our physical, mental, and emotional health.

1. **Physical fitness:** Outdoor activities offer a wide range of opportunities to engage in physical exercise. Whether it's hiking, cycling, swimming, or playing sports like tennis or soccer, these activities challenge your body and help improve cardiovascular fitness, strength, flexibility, and endurance. Outdoor activities often involve different terrains, which can provide additional challenges and benefits for your muscles and joints.

2. **Vitamin D and sun exposure:** Spending time outdoors exposes you to natural sunlight, which is a primary source of vitamin D. Vitamin D is essential for the absorption of calcium and plays a crucial role in bone health, immune function, and overall well-being. Just a few minutes of sun exposure can provide a significant boost to your vitamin D levels.

3. **Mental and emotional well-being:** Being in nature has a profound impact on our mental and emotional well-being. Studies have shown that spending time in green spaces and natural environments can reduce stress levels, improve mood, and increase feelings of happiness and relaxation. Nature has a calming effect on our minds and can help alleviate symptoms of anxiety and depression.

4. **Cognitive benefits:** Outdoor activities stimulate our senses and engage our cognitive functions. When we explore nature, we are exposed to new stimuli, such as different scents, sounds, and sights. This sensory input enhances our cognitive abilities, including attention, creativity, problem-solving, and memory. It also provides a break from constant screen time and helps improve focus and concentration.

5. **Connection with nature:** Engaging in outdoor activities allows us to connect with the natural world around us. Whether it's observing wildlife, appreciating the beauty of landscapes, or immersing ourselves in the sights and sounds of a forest or beach, these experiences foster a sense of awe, wonder, and gratitude. Connecting with nature can evoke a sense of mindfulness and promote a deeper appreciation for the world we live in.

Now, let's explore some popular outdoor activities that you can embrace:

a) **Hiking and walking:** Hiking and walking are accessible activities that allow you to explore natural trails, parks, or mountains. They provide an excellent opportunity to immerse yourself in nature, enjoy scenic views, and challenge yourself physically.

b) **Cycling:** Cycling is a fantastic way to explore your surroundings while getting a cardiovascular workout. Whether you prefer road cycling or mountain biking, it's a fun activity that can be enjoyed individually or with family and friends.

c) **Water activities:** Water activities like swimming, kayaking, paddle boarding, or surfing allow you to cool off and enjoy the benefits of being in or near water. These activities provide a full-body workout while connecting with the soothing properties of water.

d) **Team sports:** Engaging in team sports such as soccer, basketball, or volleyball in outdoor settings adds an extra element of fun and camaraderie. Gather a group of friends or join a local league to enjoy the benefits of physical activity while building social connections.

e) **Gardening:** Gardening is a fulfilling outdoor activity that combines physical movement with the joy of nurturing and growing plants. It allows you to connect with the earth, get your hands dirty, and enjoy the beauty of nature in your own backyard.

f) **Nature walks and birdwatching:** Take leisurely walks in parks or nature reserves, observing the flora and fauna around you. Birdwatching is a popular activity that encourages mindful observation and appreciation for the diverse bird species in your area.

Remember to prioritize safety while engaging in outdoor activities. Stay hydrated, protect your skin from the sun, wear appropriate footwear and clothing, and be aware of your surroundings. Always follow local guidelines and regulations regarding outdoor activities.

By embracing outdoor activities and immersing ourselves in nature, we can reap the physical, mental, and emotional benefits that contribute to our overall well-being. So, step outside, breathe in the fresh air, and embrace the wonders of the natural world around you.

Chapter 6: Overcoming Fitness Plateaus and Challenges

In any fitness journey, it's common to encounter plateaus and challenges along the way. These roadblocks can be frustrating and demotivating, but they are also opportunities for growth and improvement. This chapter focuses on overcoming fitness plateaus and challenges, providing strategies to push through obstacles, break through plateaus, and continue progressing towards your health and fitness goals.

1. Understanding Fitness Plateaus:

Fitness plateaus occur when your progress stalls, and you no longer see improvements in your performance or physical appearance. This can happen for various reasons, including a lack of variety in your workout routine, improper training techniques, insufficient recovery, or mental burnout. Understanding the underlying causes of plateaus is essential in developing effective strategies to overcome them.

Plateaus can occur in different aspects of fitness, such as strength, endurance, or body composition. For example, you may find that you can no longer increase the weight you lift or that your running speed has plateaued. It's important to recognize that plateaus are a natural part of the fitness journey and can be overcome with the right approach.

2. Assessing and Adjusting Your Routine:

The first step in overcoming plateaus is to assess your current fitness routine. Evaluate your workout program, including the exercises, intensity, duration, and frequency. Look for areas where you may have become too comfortable or repetitive. Introduce new exercises, change the order of your workouts, increase the intensity, or try different training methods to challenge your body in new ways.

Periodically reviewing and adjusting your routine is crucial for continued progress. By keeping your workouts challenging and varied, you prevent your body from adapting and hitting a plateau. Incorporating different training modalities, such as strength training, cardiovascular exercises, and flexibility work, ensures that you target different muscle groups and energy systems.

3. Periodization and Progressive Overload:

Periodization is a training technique that involves dividing your training program into different phases or cycles, each with specific goals and training methods. By implementing periodization, you can avoid stagnation and continuously challenge your body. Each phase focuses on different aspects of fitness, such as strength, power, endurance, or hypertrophy. This structured approach allows for targeted training and helps prevent plateaus.

Progressive overload is another key principle that involves gradually increasing the demands on your body over time. This can be achieved by increasing the weight, repetitions, sets, or intensity of your workouts. Progressive overload stimulates muscle growth, improves strength, and prevents adaptation. Gradually and consistently pushing your limits is essential for breaking through plateaus and achieving new levels of fitness.

4. Cross-Training and Variety:

Engaging in cross-training and incorporating variety into your workouts can help overcome plateaus. Cross-training involves participating in different types of physical activities or exercises to work different muscle groups and challenge your body in new ways. It helps prevent overuse injuries and provides mental stimulation by keeping your workouts fresh and exciting.

Try incorporating activities such as swimming, cycling, dancing, or martial arts into your routine. These activities not only add variety but also engage different muscles and energy systems. Additionally, participating in group fitness classes or team sports can provide a social aspect that adds motivation and enjoyment to your workouts.

5. Addressing Mental Blocks:

Fitness plateaus are not only physical but can also be mental. When faced with a lack of progress, it's common to experience feelings of frustration, self-doubt, or a loss of motivation. To overcome these mental blocks, it's important to reassess your goals, remind yourself of your initial motivations, and seek support from others.

Setting small, achievable goals can help you regain momentum and celebrate each milestone along the way. Focus on the process rather than the outcome, and recognize the progress you've made. Surround yourself with a supportive community or workout buddy who can provide encouragement and accountability. Additionally, finding activities that you enjoy and incorporating them into your routine can reignite your passion for fitness.

6. Prioritizing Recovery and Rest:

Proper recovery and rest are crucial for breaking through plateaus and avoiding burnout. Allow your body enough time to recover between workouts, and prioritize quality sleep to support the repair and growth of your muscles. Incorporate active recovery activities such as stretching, foam rolling, or gentle yoga to promote circulation and reduce muscle soreness.

Listening to your body and recognizing signs of overtraining or excessive fatigue is important. Give yourself permission to take rest days when needed and adjust your training intensity if necessary. Remember that progress happens during the recovery phase, not just during the workout itself.

7. Seeking Professional Guidance:

If you find yourself struggling to overcome plateaus or face specific challenges, seeking guidance from a fitness professional can be beneficial. A qualified personal trainer or fitness coach can assess your current routine, identify areas for improvement, and provide personalized recommendations.

They can introduce new training techniques, correct your form, and offer ongoing support and accountability. A professional can also help you set realistic goals and design a program tailored to your specific needs and preferences. Their expertise and guidance can help you overcome plateaus and break through barriers.

8. Staying Motivated:

Consistency is key to overcoming plateaus and achieving your fitness goals. To stay motivated, set new challenges, track your progress, and celebrate your achievements. Find a workout buddy or join fitness communities to stay connected and inspired. Keep your workouts enjoyable by incorporating your favorite activities and music.

Remind yourself of the positive changes you've experienced in your health and well-being, and maintain a positive mindset throughout your fitness journey. Reflect on how far you've come and use that as motivation to keep pushing forward. Surround yourself with supportive individuals who share your passion for fitness and can provide encouragement during challenging times.

Conclusion:

Overcoming fitness plateaus and challenges is a natural part of the fitness journey. By implementing strategies such as assessing and adjusting your routine, incorporating variety, addressing mental blocks, prioritizing recovery, seeking professional guidance, and staying motivated, you can break through plateaus and continue progressing towards your health and fitness goals.

Remember that plateaus can be temporary, and with perseverance, dedication, and a proactive mindset, you can overcome any obstacle that comes your way. Embrace the journey, celebrate your successes, and use challenges as opportunities for growth. With a resilient mindset and a willingness to adapt, you can reach new levels of fitness and achieve the healthy and vibrant life you desire.

Identifying common obstacles in maintaining a fitness routine

While embarking on a fitness journey is exciting, it's important to be aware of the potential obstacles that can hinder your progress. By identifying these common roadblocks in advance, you can develop strategies to overcome them and stay committed to your fitness routine. This section explores some of the most common obstacles individuals face when maintaining a fitness routine.

1. Lack of Time:

One of the most prevalent obstacles to maintaining a fitness routine is a perceived lack of time. Busy schedules, work commitments, family responsibilities, and other obligations can make it challenging to carve out dedicated time for exercise. However, it's essential to prioritize your health and well-being. Evaluate your daily schedule and identify time slots where you can fit in physical activity. This may involve waking up earlier, scheduling workouts during lunch breaks, or making exercise a non-negotiable part of your day.

2. Low Motivation:

Another obstacle is a lack of motivation, which can arise due to various factors such as boredom, lack of visible progress, or a feeling of being stuck in a routine. To combat this, it's crucial to find activities you enjoy and mix up your workouts to keep them interesting. Set specific goals and track your progress to stay motivated. Consider joining fitness classes or finding a workout buddy who can provide support and accountability. Remember your initial reasons for starting your fitness journey and visualize the benefits of staying committed.

3. Unrealistic Expectations:

Setting unrealistic expectations can lead to frustration and disappointment. It's important to understand that progress takes time and that results may not be immediate. Avoid comparing yourself to others and focus on your own journey. Celebrate small achievements and milestones along the way. Set realistic and achievable goals that align with your abilities and fitness level.

4. Lack of Support:

A lack of support from family, friends, or colleagues can be discouraging. Surround yourself with individuals who understand and encourage your fitness goals. Communicate with your loved ones about the importance of your fitness routine and how their support can help you stay motivated. Consider joining fitness communities or online forums where you can connect with like-minded individuals who share similar goals.

5. Injury or Health Issues:

Injuries or underlying health issues can interrupt your fitness routine. It's important to listen to your body and seek appropriate medical guidance if needed. Work with a qualified fitness professional to design a safe and effective exercise program that takes into account any existing conditions or limitations. Focus on activities that promote recovery and rehabilitation while still allowing you to maintain your fitness level.

6. Lack of Accountability:

Accountability plays a significant role in maintaining a fitness routine. Without it, it's easy to make excuses or skip workouts. Find ways to hold yourself accountable, whether it's through tracking your progress, using fitness apps, or partnering with a workout buddy. Consider working with a personal trainer or joining a group fitness class where you're expected to show up and participate.

7. Monotony and Boredom:

Doing the same workout routine day after day can become monotonous and lead to boredom. Spice up your fitness routine by trying new activities, exploring different types of exercises, or incorporating fun and challenging workouts. Set short-term goals that keep you engaged and excited about your progress. Experiment with different fitness classes, outdoor activities, or workout apps to keep your routine fresh and interesting.

Conclusion:

By identifying the common obstacles in maintaining a fitness routine, you can proactively address and overcome them. Remember that obstacles are a natural part of the journey, and with perseverance, adaptability, and a positive mindset, you can navigate through them. Seek support, stay motivated, and stay flexible in your approach. By doing so, you'll be better equipped to maintain a consistent fitness routine and achieve your health and fitness goals.

Strategies for overcoming plateaus and staying motivated

Plateaus and a lack of motivation can be challenging to navigate during a fitness journey. However, with the right strategies, you can break through plateaus and stay motivated to continue progressing towards your goals. This section explores effective strategies for overcoming plateaus and staying motivated in your fitness routine.

1. Set New Goals:

Setting new goals is an excellent way to overcome plateaus and reignite motivation. Evaluate your current progress and identify areas where you want to improve. Set specific, measurable, attainable, relevant, and time-bound (SMART) goals that challenge you and align with your fitness aspirations. By having clear objectives, you'll have a sense of purpose and direction, which can help you push through plateaus.

2. Change Up Your Routine:

Plateaus often occur due to the body adapting to a repetitive routine. Shake things up by introducing new exercises, varying the intensity, or trying different training methods. Incorporate different forms of exercise, such as strength training, cardio, HIIT workouts, or yoga, to challenge different muscle groups and energy systems. By introducing novelty into your routine, you'll stimulate your body and prevent plateaus.

3. Increase the Intensity:

Sometimes, plateaus occur because your body has adapted to your current workout intensity. To overcome this, gradually increase the intensity of your workouts. This can be done by lifting heavier weights, increasing the duration or intensity of cardio exercises, or incorporating interval training. Pushing yourself outside your comfort zone stimulates muscle growth, improves endurance, and breaks through plateaus.

4. Track Your Progress:

Keeping track of your progress is a powerful motivational tool. Use a fitness journal or a tracking app to record your workouts, set personal records, and track changes in your strength, endurance, or body composition. Seeing tangible evidence of your progress can boost your confidence and motivation, especially during plateaus. Celebrate small victories and milestones along the way to stay motivated and focused.

5. Seek Professional Guidance:

If you find yourself struggling to overcome plateaus, seeking guidance from a fitness professional can be invaluable. A qualified personal trainer or fitness coach can assess your current routine, identify areas for improvement, and provide expert recommendations. They can introduce new training techniques, correct your form, and offer ongoing support and accountability. Professional guidance can provide fresh insights and motivation to help you break through plateaus.

6. Find a Workout Buddy:

Working out with a partner or joining a fitness community can significantly enhance motivation and accountability. Find a workout buddy who shares similar goals and can provide support and encouragement. Exercising together can make workouts more enjoyable and increase your commitment. Alternatively, join group fitness classes or online fitness communities where you can connect with like-minded individuals who share similar fitness journeys.

7. Mix Up Your Environment:

Sometimes a change of environment can do wonders for your motivation. Explore new workout locations, such as outdoor parks, trails, or fitness studios. Engage in activities that allow you to enjoy nature, such as hiking, cycling, or swimming. Changing your surroundings can provide a fresh perspective, invigorate your workouts, and rekindle your enthusiasm for fitness.

8. Practice Self-Care:

Taking care of yourself physically and mentally is crucial for maintaining motivation and overcoming plateaus. Prioritize self-care activities such as getting enough sleep, managing stress, and practicing relaxation techniques like meditation or deep breathing. Nourish your body with a balanced diet, hydrate properly, and allow for adequate rest and recovery. When you take care of your overall well-being, you'll have the energy and mindset to stay motivated and push through challenges.

Conclusion:

Plateaus and a lack of motivation are common obstacles in a fitness journey, but they can be overcome with the right strategies. Set new goals, change up your routine, increase the intensity, track your progress, seek professional guidance, find a workout buddy, mix up your environment, and prioritize self-care. Remember that plateaus are temporary, and staying motivated requires perseverance and a positive mindset. By implementing these strategies, you'll be better equipped to overcome plateaus, break through barriers, and continue progressing towards your health and fitness goals.

Dealing with injuries and setbacks

Injuries and setbacks are common occurrences in a fitness journey. While they can be frustrating and discouraging, it's important to approach them with a positive mindset and develop strategies for effectively dealing with them. This section explores strategies for handling injuries and setbacks, allowing you to navigate these challenges and continue your fitness journey.

1. Listen to Your Body:

When faced with an injury or setback, it's crucial to listen to your body and give it the rest and recovery it needs. Ignoring or pushing through pain can worsen the injury and prolong your recovery time. Be mindful of any discomfort or unusual sensations during exercise, and consult a healthcare professional if necessary. Take the time to heal properly, following the guidance of medical professionals and gradually easing back into exercise when you're ready.

2. Modify Your Workout Routine:

If you're dealing with an injury, it's essential to modify your workout routine to accommodate your limitations. Consult with a healthcare professional or a qualified fitness trainer to develop a modified exercise plan that avoids exacerbating your injury. This may involve focusing on non-affected areas, incorporating low-impact exercises, or engaging in rehabilitation exercises specific to your injury. Adapting your routine ensures that you can still stay active while allowing your body to heal.

3. Seek Professional Guidance:

In cases of severe injuries or setbacks, seeking professional guidance from healthcare professionals, such as physical therapists or sports medicine specialists, is crucial. These professionals can provide targeted treatments, personalized rehabilitation plans, and expert advice on gradually returning to exercise. They can assess your injury, recommend specific exercises or therapies, and monitor your progress to ensure a safe and effective recovery.

4. Embrace Cross-Training:

During a setback or injury, cross-training can be an effective way to maintain fitness and engage different muscle groups while allowing the injured area to recover. Cross-training involves participating in alternative activities or exercises that are low-impact and don't aggravate your injury. For example, if you have a lower-body injury, you can focus on upper-body strength training or engage in low-impact activities like swimming or cycling. Cross-training keeps you active and prevents detraining while promoting overall fitness and supporting the healing process.

5. Focus on Rehabilitation and Strengthening:

Use setbacks and injuries as an opportunity to focus on rehabilitation and strengthening exercises. Work with a physical therapist or fitness professional to develop a targeted plan that addresses the affected area and helps prevent future injuries. Incorporate exercises that improve flexibility, stability, and range of motion. Gradually introduce strengthening exercises to build up the injured area and surrounding muscles. By investing in rehabilitation and strengthening, you can come back stronger and reduce the risk of re-injury.

6. Adjust Your Expectations:

Dealing with injuries or setbacks often means adjusting your expectations. Understand that recovery takes time, and progress may be slower than you'd like. Avoid comparing yourself to others or dwelling on the setbacks. Instead, focus on the small wins and improvements you make along the way. Patience and perseverance are key during this time, and maintaining a positive mindset will contribute to a successful recovery.

7. Seek Support:

Going through setbacks and injuries can be emotionally challenging. Seek support from friends, family, or a fitness community who can provide encouragement, understanding, and guidance. Share your experience and listen to others who have overcome similar obstacles. Surrounding yourself with a supportive network can help you stay motivated, maintain perspective, and navigate the emotional aspects of setbacks and injuries.

8. Learn from the Experience:

Every setback or injury can be an opportunity for growth and learning. Reflect on the possible causes of your setback and identify any areas for improvement. Assess your training techniques, equipment, form, and lifestyle habits to determine if there are any modifications you can make to prevent similar setbacks in the future. Use the setback as a chance to gain knowledge, refine your approach, and develop a more balanced and sustainable fitness routine.

Conclusion:

Injuries and setbacks are inevitable in a fitness journey, but they don't have to derail your progress. By listening to your body, modifying your routine, seeking professional guidance, embracing cross-training, focusing on rehabilitation and strengthening, adjusting your expectations, seeking support, and learning from the experience, you can effectively navigate setbacks and injuries. Remember, setbacks are temporary, and with proper care and perseverance, you can overcome them and continue working towards your health and fitness goals.

Seeking professional guidance and support

Embarking on a health and fitness journey can be overwhelming, and it's important to recognize that you don't have to navigate it alone. Seeking professional guidance and support can provide you with valuable expertise, personalized advice, and accountability to help you achieve your goals effectively and safely. This section explores the significance of seeking professional guidance and support in your health and fitness journey.

1. The Role of Fitness Professionals:

Fitness professionals, such as personal trainers, strength and conditioning coaches, and exercise physiologists, play a crucial role in guiding individuals towards their health and fitness goals. These professionals have the knowledge and expertise to design tailored workout programs, assess your fitness level, and provide guidance on proper form and technique. They can help you set realistic goals, track your progress, and modify your routine as needed. Working with a qualified fitness professional ensures that you are engaging in exercises that are appropriate for your current fitness level and are aligned with your specific goals.

2. Customized Training Programs:

One of the primary benefits of seeking professional guidance is the ability to receive customized training programs. Fitness professionals can evaluate your individual needs, taking into account factors such as your current fitness level, any pre-existing conditions or injuries, and your goals. They can design a program that optimally challenges you while ensuring your safety and progress. A customized training program takes into consideration your preferences, time constraints, and any limitations you may have, maximizing the effectiveness and enjoyment of your workouts.

3. Proper Form and Technique:

Performing exercises with correct form and technique is essential for preventing injuries and maximizing the benefits of your workouts. Fitness professionals have a keen eye for identifying and correcting improper form, ensuring that you are engaging the correct muscles and avoiding unnecessary strain. They can provide hands-on guidance, demonstrate proper technique, and offer cues to help you execute exercises effectively. Learning proper form and technique under the guidance of a professional not only minimizes the risk of injury but also allows you to make the most out of your workouts.

4. Accountability and Motivation:

Maintaining motivation and consistency in your fitness journey can be challenging, especially when faced with obstacles or a busy schedule. Seeking professional guidance provides you with built-in accountability and support. Fitness professionals can help you stay on track, provide encouragement and positive reinforcement, and hold you accountable to your goals. Knowing that you have someone to report to and receive feedback from can significantly enhance your commitment and motivation to stick to your fitness routine.

5. Safety and Injury Prevention:

Injuries can be detrimental to your progress and overall well-being. Fitness professionals are well-versed in injury prevention strategies and can help you exercise safely. They can assess any pre-existing conditions or injuries you may have and design a program that takes these factors into account. They can also provide modifications and alternatives for exercises that may aggravate your condition. Working with a professional minimizes the risk of injury and ensures that you are engaging in activities appropriate for your current fitness level.

6. Expert Advice and Education:

Fitness professionals have a wealth of knowledge when it comes to exercise science, nutrition, and overall health and wellness. They can provide you with evidence-based information, answer your questions, and debunk common fitness myths. Seeking professional guidance allows you to tap into this expertise and gain a deeper understanding of the principles behind effective training, nutrition, and lifestyle habits. By arming yourself with this knowledge, you can make informed decisions and sustain healthy habits long-term.

7. Holistic Approach to Health and Wellness:

Many fitness professionals take a holistic approach to health and wellness, recognizing the interconnectedness of physical fitness, nutrition, and mental well-being. They can provide guidance on other aspects of a healthy lifestyle, such as nutrition recommendations, stress management techniques, and sleep optimization strategies. Seeking professional guidance allows you to address your health and fitness goals from a comprehensive perspective, promoting overall well-being.

Conclusion:

Seeking professional guidance and support is a valuable investment in your health and fitness journey. Fitness professionals offer customized training programs, ensure proper form and technique, provide accountability and motivation, prioritize your safety, offer expert advice and education, and take a holistic approach to your well-being. Whether you're a beginner looking to establish a solid foundation or an experienced individual seeking to reach new heights, working with a fitness professional can greatly enhance your progress and help you achieve long-lasting results.

Chapter 7: Optimizing Sleep and Recovery

Sleep and recovery play a vital role in our overall health and well-being. In today's fast-paced world, it can be challenging to prioritize rest and recovery, but understanding their importance is crucial for optimizing our physical and mental performance. This chapter delves into the significance of sleep and recovery, exploring strategies to improve sleep quality, enhance recovery, and maximize the benefits of both.

1. The Importance of Quality Sleep:

Quality sleep is essential for maintaining optimal health. It supports various bodily functions, including immune function, hormone regulation, cognitive function, and mood regulation. Adequate sleep allows the body to repair and rejuvenate, promoting physical recovery and performance. Moreover, quality sleep is linked to better mental health, improved memory and learning, increased productivity, and overall well-being. Understanding the importance of sleep and prioritizing its quality sets the foundation for enhanced performance in all aspects of life.

2. Sleep Hygiene Practices:

To optimize sleep, it's crucial to establish healthy sleep hygiene practices. These practices involve creating a sleep-friendly environment, implementing a consistent sleep schedule, and adopting pre-sleep routines that promote relaxation. Managing exposure to light, keeping the bedroom cool and quiet, and avoiding stimulating activities or electronic devices before bedtime can improve sleep quality. Establishing a relaxing routine, such as reading, meditating, or taking a warm bath, signals the body to prepare for sleep. By adopting these sleep hygiene practices, you can enhance your ability to fall asleep faster and enjoy more restful sleep.

3. Strategies for Better Sleep:

In addition to sleep hygiene practices, several strategies can help improve sleep quality. Regular exercise during the day promotes better sleep, but it's important to avoid vigorous exercise close to bedtime. Managing stress through relaxation techniques like deep breathing, progressive muscle relaxation, or journaling can also contribute to better sleep. Additionally, establishing a regular sleep schedule, including consistent wake-up and bedtime routines, helps regulate the body's internal clock and promotes a more balanced sleep-wake cycle. Experimenting with different sleep positions, investing in a comfortable mattress and pillows, and creating a sleep-inducing atmosphere can also enhance sleep quality.

4. The Role of Nutrition in Sleep:

Nutrition plays a significant role in sleep quality. Consuming a balanced diet that includes foods rich in sleep-supporting nutrients, such as magnesium, tryptophan, and melatonin, can help promote better sleep. Avoiding large meals, caffeine, and alcohol close to bedtime can also improve sleep quality. It's important to establish a healthy eating pattern that supports sleep, incorporating nutrient-dense foods while being mindful of timing and portion sizes. Creating a nighttime routine that includes a light, sleep-supporting snack can also aid in promoting relaxation and supporting a good night's sleep.

5. Active Recovery Strategies:

Recovery is not just about sleep; it also involves active strategies to promote physical and mental rejuvenation. Active recovery techniques, such as gentle stretching, foam rolling, or low-impact activities like yoga or swimming, can help improve circulation, reduce muscle soreness, and enhance flexibility. Engaging in active recovery promotes relaxation, reduces stress, and aids in the removal of metabolic waste from the muscles, facilitating faster recovery between workouts.

6. Rest and Relaxation Techniques:

Aside from physical recovery, incorporating rest and relaxation techniques into your routine is essential for mental and emotional well-being. Techniques like meditation, deep breathing exercises, mindfulness practices, and relaxation exercises can reduce stress, calm the mind, and improve overall relaxation. Taking time for self-care activities, such as reading, listening to calming music, or engaging in hobbies, helps recharge and rejuvenate the mind, fostering a sense of balance and well-being.

Conclusion:

Optimizing sleep and recovery is crucial for achieving optimal health, performance, and well-being. By understanding the importance of quality sleep, implementing sleep hygiene practices, adopting strategies for better sleep, considering the role of nutrition, embracing active recovery techniques, and incorporating rest and relaxation into our routines, we can effectively optimize sleep and recovery. Prioritizing these aspects of our lives empowers us to perform at our best, maintain physical and mental health, and lead a fulfilling and balanced lifestyle.

Understanding the importance of quality sleep

Sleep is an essential biological process that is crucial for our overall health and well-being. It is during sleep that our bodies and minds undergo repair, restoration, and consolidation of information. In this section, we will explore the significance of quality sleep and how it impacts various aspects of our lives.

1. Physical Health:

Quality sleep plays a vital role in maintaining and promoting physical health. During sleep, our bodies engage in important restorative processes, such as tissue repair, muscle growth, and hormone regulation. Sufficient and restful sleep supports immune function, helping to defend against infections and reduce the risk of chronic diseases such as diabetes, cardiovascular diseases, and obesity. Additionally, sleep is closely linked to healthy metabolism, appetite regulation, and weight management. Lack of quality sleep has been associated with an increased risk of weight gain and obesity due to hormonal imbalances that affect appetite control.

2. Cognitive Function:

Sleep is closely intertwined with cognitive function and brain health. Adequate sleep is crucial for optimal cognitive performance, including attention, concentration, memory consolidation, and learning. During sleep, the brain consolidates and organizes information gathered throughout the day, strengthening neural connections and enhancing memory recall. Getting enough sleep improves problem-solving abilities, creativity, and decision-making skills. On the other hand, sleep deprivation impairs cognitive function, leading to difficulties in focus, attention, and memory retrieval.

3. Emotional Well-being:

Sleep has a profound impact on our emotional well-being. Quality sleep contributes to emotional regulation, resilience, and overall mental health. Sufficient sleep helps regulate mood, reducing the risk of mood disorders such as anxiety and depression. When we lack quality sleep, we may experience increased irritability, mood swings, and heightened emotional reactivity. Chronic sleep deprivation has also been associated with an increased risk of developing mental health disorders and a decrease in overall psychological well-being.

4. Energy and Productivity:

Quality sleep is essential for maintaining optimal energy levels and promoting productivity. When we get enough sleep, we wake up feeling refreshed and energized, ready to take on the day's tasks. Good sleep supports sustained attention, mental clarity, and problem-solving abilities, allowing us to perform at our best in work, school, and daily activities. In contrast, insufficient or poor-quality sleep can lead to daytime sleepiness, fatigue, decreased focus, and reduced productivity.

5. Physical Performance:

For individuals engaged in physical activities or sports, quality sleep is crucial for optimal performance and recovery. During sleep, the body repairs and rebuilds muscles, restores energy stores, and regulates hormonal balance. Athletes who prioritize sleep experience improved reaction times, faster muscle recovery, enhanced endurance, and better overall performance. Conversely, inadequate sleep can impair coordination, reaction times, and muscle recovery, increasing the risk of injuries and compromising athletic performance.

Conclusion:

Understanding the importance of quality sleep is fundamental to prioritizing our overall health and well-being. By recognizing the profound impact that sleep has on physical health, cognitive function, emotional well-being, energy levels, and physical performance, we can make conscious efforts to improve our sleep habits. Establishing a consistent sleep routine, creating a sleep-friendly environment, practicing relaxation techniques, and adopting healthy sleep hygiene practices can significantly enhance the quality and duration of our sleep, leading to a healthier, happier, and more productive life.

Developing healthy sleep habits and a bedtime routine

Establishing healthy sleep habits and a consistent bedtime routine is essential for promoting quality sleep and optimizing our overall well-being. In this section, we will explore the key components of healthy sleep habits and provide practical tips for developing an effective bedtime routine.

1. Consistent Sleep Schedule:

Maintaining a consistent sleep schedule is crucial for regulating your body's internal clock, also known as the circadian rhythm. Try to go to bed and wake up at the same time every day, even on weekends. This helps establish a regular sleep-wake cycle, allowing your body to anticipate and prepare for sleep. Consistency in sleep schedule enhances the quality and efficiency of sleep, ensuring you feel refreshed and energized upon waking.

2. Create a Sleep-Friendly Environment:

Your sleep environment plays a significant role in the quality of your sleep. Make your bedroom a comfortable and relaxing space that promotes sleep. Ensure the room is cool, dark, and quiet. Consider using blackout curtains, earplugs, or a white noise machine to block out any disruptive external stimuli. Invest in a comfortable mattress, pillows, and bedding that provide proper support and comfort. Remove electronic devices that emit blue light, as it can interfere with your body's natural sleep-wake cycle.

3. Establish a Wind-Down Routine:

A bedtime routine helps signal to your body that it's time to relax and prepare for sleep. Designate a period before bed for winding down and engaging in relaxing activities. This can include reading a book, taking a warm bath or shower, practicing gentle stretching or yoga, or listening to calming music. Avoid stimulating activities, such as intense exercise or using electronic devices, as they can interfere with your ability to fall asleep.

4. Limit Stimulants and Caffeine Intake:

Be mindful of your consumption of stimulants, especially in the hours leading up to bedtime. Avoid consuming caffeine, nicotine, and alcohol, as they can disrupt your sleep patterns and make it harder to fall asleep. Instead, opt for soothing herbal teas or warm milk, which can promote relaxation and aid in sleep.

5. Practice Relaxation Techniques:

Incorporating relaxation techniques into your bedtime routine can help calm your mind and prepare your body for sleep. Deep breathing exercises, progressive muscle relaxation, and mindfulness meditation are effective techniques to reduce stress and promote a sense of relaxation. These practices help quiet racing thoughts, alleviate anxiety, and induce a state of calm conducive to sleep.

6. Limit Napping:

If you struggle with falling asleep or staying asleep at night, it may be helpful to limit daytime napping. Short power naps of around 20-30 minutes can provide a quick energy boost, but longer or late-afternoon naps can interfere with your ability to sleep at night. If you do need to nap, try to do so earlier in the day and keep it brief.

7. Create a Bedtime Ritual:

Establishing a consistent bedtime ritual can condition your body and mind to prepare for sleep. This can involve activities such as brushing your teeth, washing your face, or reading a few pages of a book. Engaging in the same sequence of activities each night can create a sense of familiarity and cue your body that it's time to sleep.

Conclusion:

Developing healthy sleep habits and a bedtime routine is a valuable investment in your overall well-being. By prioritizing a consistent sleep schedule, creating a sleep-friendly environment, establishing a wind-down routine, limiting stimulants, practicing relaxation techniques, and cultivating a bedtime ritual, you can optimize the quality and duration of your sleep. These habits and routines promote restful sleep, enhance daytime energy and productivity, and contribute to your overall physical and mental health. Remember, it may take time to establish these habits, so be patient with yourself and remain consistent in your efforts.

Enhancing recovery through proper nutrition and rest

Proper nutrition and rest play a vital role in optimizing recovery from physical activity, promoting muscle repair, reducing inflammation, and replenishing energy stores. In this section, we will explore the importance of nutrition and rest in recovery and provide strategies for maximizing their benefits.

1. Nutrition for Recovery:

Macronutrients:

Protein: Consuming an adequate amount of protein is crucial for muscle repair and growth. Include lean sources of protein such as chicken, fish, tofu, legumes, and dairy products in your post-workout meals.

Carbohydrates: Carbohydrates are the primary source of energy for your body. Consuming complex carbohydrates such as whole grains, fruits, and vegetables helps replenish glycogen stores and supports recovery.

Fats: Healthy fats, such as avocados, nuts, seeds, and olive oil, provide essential nutrients and help reduce inflammation.

Micronutrients:

Vitamins and Minerals: Ensure you are getting a variety of vitamins and minerals through a balanced diet or supplementation. Key nutrients for recovery include vitamin C, vitamin E, zinc, magnesium, and iron.

Hydration:

Proper hydration is essential for optimal recovery. Drink plenty of water throughout the day, and especially after workouts, to replace fluids lost through sweat. Consider adding electrolytes to your water or consuming sports drinks for longer or intense exercise sessions.

2. Rest and Sleep for Recovery:

Active Rest: Engage in active rest days, where you participate in low-intensity activities such as walking, stretching, or yoga. Active rest promotes blood circulation, helps prevent muscle stiffness, and aids in recovery.

Sleep: Quality sleep is crucial for recovery. Aim for 7-9 hours of uninterrupted sleep each night. During sleep, your body releases growth hormone, repairs tissues, and restores energy levels. Create a conducive sleep environment and follow a consistent sleep routine.

3. Recovery Techniques:

Foam Rolling and Stretching: Incorporate foam rolling and stretching exercises into your post-workout routine. These techniques help release muscle tension, improve flexibility, and reduce muscle soreness.

Cold and Heat Therapy: Alternating between cold and heat therapy, such as ice baths or hot showers, can help reduce inflammation, soothe muscles, and enhance recovery.

Massage and Bodywork: Consider regular massages or other bodywork techniques to relax muscles, improve blood circulation, and aid in recovery.

4. Listen to Your Body:

 Pay attention to your body's signals and adjust your training intensity, volume, and recovery strategies accordingly. Rest when needed, and avoid pushing through pain or fatigue, as it may lead to injury or prolonged recovery.

Conclusion:

Proper nutrition and rest are essential components of an effective recovery plan. By fueling your body with the right nutrients, staying hydrated, prioritizing quality sleep, incorporating active rest, and utilizing recovery techniques, you can enhance your body's ability to repair, rebuild, and adapt to physical activity. Remember, every individual is unique, so it's important to listen to your body's needs and make adjustments as necessary to optimize your recovery process.

Exploring relaxation techniques for better sleep

Incorporating relaxation techniques into your bedtime routine can help promote better sleep by calming the mind, reducing stress, and preparing your body for a restful night. In this section, we will explore various relaxation techniques that you can explore to improve the quality of your sleep.

1. Deep Breathing Exercises:

Deep breathing exercises are a simple yet effective way to relax the body and mind before sleep. Try the following technique:

- Lie down comfortably in bed and close your eyes.

- Inhale deeply through your nose, filling your abdomen with air.

- Exhale slowly through your mouth, releasing all the air and letting go of tension.

- Repeat this deep breathing pattern, focusing on your breath and allowing your body to relax with each exhale.

2. Progressive Muscle Relaxation (PMR):

Progressive Muscle Relaxation involves tensing and then relaxing each muscle group in your body, promoting a deep state of relaxation. Follow these steps:

- Start with your toes and progressively work your way up, tensing and then relaxing each muscle group.

- Take a deep breath as you tense the muscles, hold for a few seconds, and then release the tension as you exhale.

- Focus on the sensation of relaxation as the tension leaves your muscles.

3. Guided Imagery:

Guided imagery involves using your imagination to create a peaceful and calming mental image, promoting relaxation and reducing stress. You can use pre-recorded guided imagery audios or create your own imagery by:

- Closing your eyes and visualizing a serene and tranquil setting, such as a beach or a peaceful garden.
- Engaging all your senses to immerse yourself in the imaginary environment, imagining the sights, sounds, smells, and sensations.

4. Aromatherapy:

Aromatherapy involves using scents to promote relaxation and better sleep. Some calming scents include lavender, chamomile, jasmine, and sandalwood. You can use essential oils in various ways:

- Diffuse essential oils in your bedroom before sleep.
- Add a few drops of essential oil to a warm bath or use them in a pre-bedtime massage oil.

5. Sleep-Friendly Environment:

Creating a sleep-friendly environment can enhance relaxation and promote better sleep. Consider the following tips:

- Keep your bedroom cool, dark, and quiet.
- Use blackout curtains or an eye mask to block out light.
- Use earplugs or a white noise machine to mask external noises.
- Remove electronic devices or place them on "do not disturb" mode to minimize distractions.

6. Mindfulness Meditation:

Mindfulness meditation involves focusing your attention on the present moment, allowing thoughts and sensations to come and go without judgment. Practicing mindfulness meditation before sleep can help quiet the mind and induce a state of relaxation. You can start with these steps:

- Find a comfortable position, either sitting or lying down.
- Focus your attention on your breath, observing each inhalation and exhalation.
- If thoughts arise, gently acknowledge them and let them go, returning your focus to your breath.

Conclusion:

Exploring relaxation techniques can greatly contribute to better sleep by reducing stress, calming the mind, and preparing the body for rest. Incorporate deep breathing exercises, progressive muscle relaxation, guided imagery, aromatherapy, mindfulness meditation, and create a sleep-friendly environment to enhance relaxation before bedtime. Experiment with different techniques and find what works best for you, establishing a consistent routine that promotes relaxation and prepares you for a restful night's sleep. Remember, the goal is to create a tranquil and peaceful environment that allows you to let go of the day's stresses and promote deep relaxation for a rejuvenating sleep experience.

Chapter 8: Maintaining Long-Term Success

Achieving your health and fitness goals is a significant accomplishment, but the journey doesn't end there. Sustaining long-term success requires commitment, consistency, and a proactive approach to your overall well-being. In this chapter, we will explore key strategies and habits that will help you maintain your progress and continue living a healthy and fit lifestyle. From mindset and goal-setting to accountability and adapting to change, this chapter will provide valuable insights to support your ongoing success.

1. Developing a Growth Mindset:

To maintain long-term success, it's essential to cultivate a growth mindset. Embrace the belief that you have the ability to continuously improve and grow in your health and fitness journey. Adopt a positive and resilient attitude, viewing setbacks as opportunities for learning and growth. Challenge yourself to step outside your comfort zone, embrace new challenges, and strive for ongoing personal development.

2. Refining Your Goals:

Regularly reassess and refine your goals to ensure they align with your evolving aspirations and priorities. Set specific, measurable, achievable, relevant, and time-bound (SMART) goals that provide you with clear direction and motivation. Break down your long-term goals into smaller, manageable milestones to celebrate your achievements along the way. Regularly evaluate your progress, make necessary adjustments, and set new goals to maintain forward momentum.

3. Tracking Your Progress:

Implement effective tracking methods to monitor your progress and maintain accountability. Keep a workout journal or use fitness tracking apps to record your exercise routines, nutrition intake, and other relevant metrics. Tracking your progress helps you stay focused, identify patterns, and make informed adjustments to your habits and routines. Celebrate your milestones and use your progress as a source of motivation to keep moving forward.

4. Embracing a Balanced Lifestyle:

Sustaining long-term success goes beyond fitness and nutrition. It involves embracing a balanced and holistic lifestyle. Prioritize self-care activities, such as relaxation techniques, hobbies, and quality time with loved ones. Seek a healthy work-life balance that allows you to manage stress effectively and prioritize your well-being. Remember that true success is achieved when you feel fulfilled in all areas of your life.

5. Adapting to Change:

Life is dynamic, and adapting to change is crucial for maintaining long-term success. Embrace flexibility and openness to adjust your routines, goals, and strategies as circumstances evolve. Whether it's a change in your schedule, new responsibilities, or unexpected challenges, be adaptable and find creative ways to integrate health and fitness into your life. Seek support from your support system, seek professional guidance, and stay resilient in the face of change.

6. Building a Supportive Network:

Surround yourself with like-minded individuals who share similar health and fitness goals. Cultivate a supportive network that encourages and motivates you on your journey. This can be through joining fitness communities, participating in group activities, or connecting with individuals who inspire you. Having a support system not only provides accountability but also offers a sense of camaraderie and shared experiences.

7. Self-Care and Recovery:

Prioritize self-care and recovery to avoid burnout and sustain long-term success. Listen to your body's signals and give yourself permission to rest when needed. Incorporate active recovery activities such as gentle stretching, yoga, or low-intensity workouts into your routine. Practice stress-management techniques, engage in activities that bring you joy, and prioritize quality sleep to support your overall well-being.

Conclusion:

Maintaining long-term success requires a proactive and multifaceted approach. By cultivating a growth mindset, refining your goals, tracking your progress, embracing a balanced lifestyle, adapting to change, building a supportive network, and prioritizing self-care and recovery, you can create a sustainable foundation for ongoing health and fitness success. Remember that your journey is unique, and it's essential to find strategies that resonate with you personally. Stay committed, stay motivated, and embrace the continuous process of growth and self-improvement as you maintain your health and fitness for the long term.

Strategies for staying consistent with health and fitness goals

Consistency is key when it comes to achieving and maintaining your health and fitness goals. It is the daily commitment to healthy habits and routines that ultimately leads to long-term success. In this section, we will explore effective strategies to help you stay consistent and on track with your health and fitness goals.

1. Establish a Routine:

Creating a consistent routine is essential for staying on track with your health and fitness goals. Set specific times for your workouts and meals, making them non-negotiable appointments in your schedule. By establishing a routine, you eliminate decision fatigue and make it easier to prioritize your health and fitness consistently.

2. Set Realistic and Achievable Goals:

Setting realistic and achievable goals is crucial for maintaining consistency. Break down your long-term goals into smaller, attainable milestones. This not only gives you a sense of accomplishment but also allows you to stay motivated and committed. Celebrate each milestone, and use them as stepping stones towards your larger objectives.

3. Find Activities You Enjoy:

One of the most effective ways to stay consistent with your health and fitness goals is to engage in activities you genuinely enjoy. Whether it's dancing, hiking, cycling, or playing a sport, find activities that bring you joy and make you look forward to being active. When you enjoy what you're doing, it becomes easier to stay consistent and maintain a lifelong commitment.

4. Build a Support System:

Surrounding yourself with a supportive network can significantly impact your consistency. Seek out like-minded individuals who share similar health and fitness goals. This can be friends, family, or joining fitness communities both online and offline. Having a support system provides accountability, encouragement, and a sense of community, making it easier to stay consistent and motivated.

5. Track Your Progress:

Monitoring your progress is a powerful tool for maintaining consistency. Keep a record of your workouts, nutrition, and measurements. This allows you to see how far you've come and provides tangible evidence of your efforts. Use fitness tracking apps, journals, or spreadsheets to track your progress and celebrate your achievements along the way.

6. Plan and Prepare Ahead:

Planning and preparation are key to maintaining consistency. Set aside time each week to plan your meals, schedule your workouts, and make a grocery list. By having a plan in place, you eliminate guesswork and reduce the likelihood of making unhealthy choices due to lack of preparation. Prepare healthy meals in advance, pack your gym bag the night before, and create an environment that supports your health and fitness goals.

7. Practice Self-Care:

Taking care of yourself both physically and mentally is crucial for consistency. Prioritize self-care activities that help you relax, recharge, and reduce stress. This can include activities like meditation, deep breathing exercises, taking baths, or engaging in hobbies that bring you joy. When you prioritize self-care, you enhance your overall well-being, making it easier to stay consistent with your health and fitness goals.

8. Stay Flexible and Adapt:

Life is unpredictable, and staying consistent requires adaptability. Be prepared for unexpected challenges or changes in your schedule. Instead of viewing them as setbacks, find creative solutions to keep moving forward. If you miss a workout, find alternative ways to be active. If your schedule changes, adjust your routine accordingly. Being flexible and adaptable allows you to maintain consistency despite life's curveballs.

Conclusion:

Staying consistent with your health and fitness goals is a continuous journey that requires commitment, dedication, and a proactive approach. By establishing a routine, setting realistic goals, finding activities you enjoy, building a support system, tracking your progress, planning ahead, practicing self-care, and staying flexible, you can cultivate a lifestyle of consistency. Remember, consistency is not about perfection but about making conscious choices every day that align with your health and fitness goals.

Setting realistic expectations and celebrating milestones

Setting realistic expectations and celebrating milestones are essential components of maintaining consistency and long-term success in your health and fitness journey. It's important to establish a healthy mindset that acknowledges progress and celebrates achievements along the way. In this section, we will explore strategies for setting realistic expectations and ways to celebrate milestones, fostering motivation and continued commitment to your health and fitness goals.

1. Set Realistic and Attainable Goals:

When it comes to setting expectations, it's crucial to be realistic and attainable. Unrealistic goals can lead to frustration and demotivation. Take into consideration your current fitness level, lifestyle, and any limitations you may have. Set goals that challenge you but are within your reach. This allows for a sense of accomplishment and sets the stage for sustainable progress.

2. Break Down Long-Term Goals:

Long-term goals can feel overwhelming, especially when progress is not immediately visible. Break down your long-term goals into smaller, manageable milestones. This provides you with a clear roadmap and allows you to celebrate achievements along the way. Each milestone reached serves as a source of motivation and keeps you engaged in the process.

3. Focus on Non-Scale Victories:

While the scale is one way to measure progress, it's important to broaden your perspective and focus on non-scale victories as well. Celebrate improvements in strength, endurance, flexibility, and overall well-being. Pay attention to how your clothes fit, how you feel mentally and emotionally, and the positive changes you notice in your daily life. Recognize and appreciate these non-scale victories as meaningful milestones on your journey.

4. Embrace the Process:

Achieving lasting results takes time, consistency, and effort. Embrace the process and shift your focus from solely outcome-based goals to the daily habits and behaviors that support your overall well-being. Celebrate the small wins, such as completing a challenging workout or sticking to a healthy eating plan for a week. Emphasize the positive changes you are making in your lifestyle, as these ultimately contribute to your long-term success.

5. Practice Gratitude and Self-Reflection:

Take moments to reflect on your progress and express gratitude for how far you've come. Acknowledge the effort, dedication, and commitment you have put into your health and fitness journey. Celebrate your achievements by expressing gratitude for the opportunities, resources, and support that have contributed to your success. Practicing gratitude cultivates a positive mindset and reinforces your motivation to continue.

6. Reward Yourself:

Rewarding yourself for reaching milestones can be a powerful motivator. Choose rewards that align with your health and fitness goals, such as treating yourself to a massage, buying new workout gear, or indulging in a non-food-related reward. These rewards serve as tangible reminders of your progress and provide additional motivation to stay consistent.

7. Share Your Success:

Share your success and milestones with others. Celebrate your achievements with friends, family, or your support network. Their encouragement and positive reinforcement can amplify your sense of accomplishment and motivate you to keep pushing forward. Sharing your journey also allows you to inspire and motivate others, creating a positive ripple effect within your community.

8. Learn from Setbacks:

It's important to recognize that setbacks and challenges are a normal part of any journey. Instead of becoming discouraged, view setbacks as opportunities for growth and learning. Reflect on what you can do differently or adjust in your approach. By embracing setbacks as learning experiences, you can navigate them with resilience and continue moving forward.

Conclusion:

Setting realistic expectations and celebrating milestones are essential for maintaining motivation, commitment, and long-term success in your health and fitness journey. By setting attainable goals, breaking them down into smaller milestones, focusing on non-scale victories, embracing the process, practicing gratitude, rewarding yourself, sharing your success, and learning from setbacks, you create a positive and sustainable mindset. Remember, progress is a journey, and each milestone reached is a testament to your dedication and perseverance. Celebrate your achievements and continue striving for a healthier and fitter you.

Creating a support system and finding accountability partners

Building a support system and finding accountability partners are crucial components of maintaining long-term success in your health and fitness journey. Having a network of individuals who understand and support your goals can provide motivation, guidance, and encouragement during challenging times. In this section, we will explore strategies for creating a support system and finding accountability partners to help you stay on track and achieve your health and fitness goals.

1. Identify Your Needs:

Before seeking a support system or accountability partners, it's important to identify your specific needs. Determine the type of support and accountability that would benefit you most. Are you looking for someone to exercise with, share nutritional tips, or provide emotional support? Understanding your needs will help you find the right individuals or groups to support you on your journey.

Engage in Fitness Communities:

Joining fitness communities, whether in-person or online, is a great way to find like-minded individuals who share similar health and fitness goals. These communities often provide a supportive and encouraging environment where you can connect with others, share experiences, and seek advice. Look for fitness classes, local fitness groups, or online forums that align with your interests.

3. Seek Support from Friends and Family:

Reach out to friends and family members who are supportive of your health and fitness goals. Share your aspirations with them and explain the importance of their support. They can provide encouragement, accountability, and join you in activities such as workouts or healthy meal planning. Having the support of loved ones can make a significant difference in your journey.

4. Find an Accountability Partner:

An accountability partner is someone who shares similar goals and holds you accountable for your actions. They can be a friend, family member, or even a colleague. Choose someone who is committed to their own health and fitness journey and is willing to provide support and hold you accountable. Regular check-ins, shared progress updates, and joint activities can help keep you both motivated and accountable.

5. Join Online Support Groups:

The online world offers a wealth of support groups and communities dedicated to health and fitness. Look for social media groups, forums, or apps that focus on specific goals or interests. These platforms provide opportunities to connect with individuals who are on a similar path, offering virtual support, advice, and motivation. Participating in these groups can be a source of inspiration and accountability.

3. Consider Professional Support:

Sometimes, seeking professional support can be beneficial in creating a solid support system. Working with a personal trainer, nutritionist, or health coach can provide expert guidance, personalized advice, and a structured approach to your health and fitness journey. These professionals can help you set realistic goals, monitor your progress, and provide valuable insights and motivation.

4. Engage in Group Activities:

Participating in group activities, such as fitness classes, sports teams, or exercise challenges, can help you build a support system while enjoying the camaraderie of others. These activities provide opportunities to connect with individuals who share similar interests and goals. You can cheer each other on, celebrate achievements, and create a sense of accountability within the group. 8. Be a Supportive Partner: Building a support system is not only about receiving support but also about providing it to others. Be a supportive partner to someone else on their health and fitness journey. Share your knowledge, offer encouragement, and celebrate their achievements. By being a source of support to others, you reinforce your own commitment and create a reciprocal relationship.

Conclusion:

Creating a support system and finding accountability partners are crucial steps in maintaining long-term success in your health and fitness journey. Surrounding yourself with individuals who understand and support your goals provides motivation, guidance, and encouragement when faced with challenges. Whether through fitness communities, friends and family, online groups, or professional support, a solid support system will help you stay on track, celebrate your victories, and navigate obstacles with greater resilience. Embrace the power of a support system and accountability partners as you continue your journey towards a healthier and fitter lifestyle.

Embracing a holistic approach to overall wellness

Top of Form

When it comes to achieving and maintaining long-term success in your health and fitness journey, adopting a holistic approach to overall wellness is key. Holistic wellness encompasses not only physical health but also mental, emotional, and spiritual well-being. It recognizes the interconnectedness of different aspects of our lives and emphasizes the importance of balance and harmony. In this section, we will explore the significance of embracing a holistic approach to overall wellness and how it can contribute to your health and fitness goals.

1. Nurturing Physical Health:

Physical health is a fundamental aspect of holistic wellness. It involves engaging in regular exercise, eating a nutritious diet, and taking care of your body's physical needs. Prioritize activities that strengthen your cardiovascular system, build muscular strength, and enhance flexibility. Pay attention to the quality and quantity of food you consume, ensuring a balanced and nourishing diet. Taking care of your physical health provides the foundation for overall well-being.

2. Cultivating Mental and Emotional Well-Being:

A holistic approach to wellness recognizes the importance of mental and emotional well-being. Engage in activities that promote mental clarity, reduce stress, and enhance emotional resilience. Practice mindfulness and meditation to cultivate a calm and centered mind. Seek ways to manage stress effectively, such as engaging in hobbies, spending time in nature, or engaging in creative outlets. Taking care of your mental and emotional health supports your overall wellness and positively impacts your health and fitness journey.

3. Nourishing Your Spirituality:

Spirituality plays a significant role in holistic wellness. It involves connecting with your inner self, finding meaning and purpose in life, and fostering a sense of connection to something greater than yourself. Explore practices that align with your spiritual beliefs, such as meditation, prayer, journaling, or spending time in nature. Nurturing your spirituality can provide a sense of grounding, peace, and fulfillment.

4. Cultivating Healthy Relationships:

Healthy relationships contribute to overall wellness. Surround yourself with supportive and positive individuals who uplift and inspire you. Foster meaningful connections and cultivate open and honest communication with your loved ones. Engage in activities that promote bonding and create shared experiences. Building and maintaining healthy relationships nourishes your emotional well-being and provides a solid support system for your health and fitness journey.

5. Prioritizing Self-Care:

Self-care is a vital aspect of holistic wellness. It involves intentionally setting aside time for activities that rejuvenate and restore your energy. Engage in self-care practices that resonate with you, such as taking relaxing baths, practicing self-reflection, indulging in hobbies, or getting quality sleep. Prioritizing self-care allows you to recharge, reduce stress, and maintain balance in your life.

6. Finding Work-Life Balance:

Achieving work-life balance is crucial for holistic wellness. Strive to create a harmonious integration between your professional and personal life. Set boundaries, prioritize self-care, and allocate time for activities that bring you joy and fulfillment outside of work. Finding a balance between work and other aspects of your life enhances your overall well-being and supports your health and fitness goals.

7. Practicing Gratitude:

Cultivating gratitude is an integral part of a holistic approach to wellness. Take time each day to reflect on and appreciate the blessings and positive aspects of your life. Practice gratitude journaling, express gratitude to others, or engage in gratitude rituals that resonate with you. Practicing gratitude cultivates a positive mindset, enhances overall well-being, and strengthens your resilience on your health and fitness journey.

Conclusion:

Embracing a holistic approach to overall wellness is essential for long-term success in your health and fitness journey. By nurturing your physical health, cultivating mental and emotional well-being, nourishing your spirituality, prioritizing healthy relationships, practicing self-care, finding work -life balance, and cultivating gratitude, you create a solid foundation for a healthy and fulfilling life. Adopting a holistic mindset allows you to address all aspects of your well-being and leads to a more balanced, vibrant, and sustainable approach to health and fitness.

Conclusion:

In conclusion, this book on health and fitness has covered a wide range of topics to help you understand the importance of maintaining a healthy lifestyle. From the foundations of health and fitness to designing personalized workout plans, optimizing nutrition, managing stress and emotions, integrating physical activity into everyday life, overcoming challenges, and prioritizing sleep and recovery, each chapter has provided valuable insights and practical strategies.

By emphasizing the significance of health and fitness in modern society, setting goals, and creating a healthy mindset, you have learned the essential building blocks for embarking on a successful health and fitness journey. Understanding the impact of exercise on physical and mental well-being has highlighted the importance of incorporating regular physical activity into your routine.

Recognizing the role of nutrition in maintaining optimal health has provided insights into the significance of macronutrients, micronutrients, and balanced meal planning. Strategies for portion control and mindful eating have equipped you with the tools to maintain a healthy relationship with food.

Exploring the importance of sleep and stress management has underscored the significance of quality sleep and relaxation techniques for overall wellness. Additionally, the chapter on the mind-body connection has highlighted the impact of emotions and stress on health and provided techniques for managing them effectively.

The chapter on building a solid fitness routine has provided guidance on assessing your current fitness level, setting realistic goals, and designing personalized workout plans that include cardiovascular exercises, strength training, flexibility exercises, and interval training for optimal results.

Understanding the significance of a holistic approach to overall wellness has emphasized the importance of nurturing physical health, cultivating mental and emotional well-being, nourishing spirituality, prioritizing healthy relationships, practicing self-care, finding work-life balance, and practicing gratitude.

Finally, the chapter on maintaining long-term success has explored strategies for staying consistent with health and fitness goals, setting realistic expectations, celebrating milestones, creating a support system, finding accountability partners, and embracing a holistic approach to wellness.

By incorporating the knowledge and implementing the strategies outlined in this book, you are well-equipped to embark on your health and fitness journey with confidence and success. Remember, the key lies in consistency, perseverance, and a commitment to your well-being. With each step forward, you are actively investing in a healthier, happier, and more fulfilling life.

Recap of key concepts and takeaways

Throughout this book on health and fitness, we have explored various topics and provided valuable insights and strategies to help you lead a healthier and more fulfilling life. Let's recap some of the key concepts and takeaways:

Health and Fitness in Modern Society:

We emphasized the importance of health and fitness in today's society, considering the physical, mental, and emotional benefits they offer.

Setting Goals and Creating a Healthy Mindset:

We discussed the significance of setting clear and achievable goals, as well as cultivating a positive and resilient mindset to overcome challenges.

The Impact of Exercise on Physical and Mental Well-being:

We delved into how regular exercise can improve cardiovascular health, increase strength and muscle development, enhance flexibility, and boost mental well-being.

The Role of Nutrition in Maintaining Optimal Health:

We explored the importance of macronutrients (carbohydrates, proteins, and fats) and micronutrients (vitamins and minerals) in a balanced diet, as well as the creation of personalized meal plans and strategies for portion control.

The Importance of Sleep and Stress Management in Overall Wellness:

We discussed the significance of quality sleep and explored techniques for relaxation, stress management, and improving sleep habits.

Building a Solid Fitness Routine:

We covered topics such as assessing your fitness level, setting realistic goals, designing personalized workout plans that incorporate cardiovascular exercises, strength training, flexibility exercises, and interval training.

Mastering Nutritional Balance:

We highlighted the importance of understanding macronutrients and their functions, as well as the significance of micronutrients in a healthy diet. We also explored creating balanced meal plans.

Mind-Body Connection:

Managing Stress and Emotions: We explored the mind-body connection and its impact on health, techniques for stress management and relaxation (excluding yoga), the power of meditation and mindfulness practices, and emotional well-being.

Integrating Physical Activity into Everyday Life:

We discussed incorporating exercise into a busy schedule, active commuting, making fitness a family affair, and embracing outdoor activities for the benefits of nature.

Overcoming Fitness Plateaus and Challenges:

We covered identifying common obstacles in maintaining a fitness routine, strategies for overcoming plateaus and staying motivated, dealing with injuries and setbacks, and seeking professional guidance and support.

Optimizing Sleep and Recovery:

We emphasized the importance of quality sleep, developing healthy sleep habits and a bedtime routine, enhancing recovery through nutrition and rest, and exploring relaxation techniques for better sleep.

Maintaining Long-Term Success:

We discussed strategies for staying consistent with health and fitness goals, setting realistic expectations, celebrating milestones, creating a support system, finding accountability partners, and embracing a holistic approach to overall wellness.

By understanding and implementing these key concepts and takeaways, you are empowered to make positive changes in your life, improve your overall well-being, and achieve long-term success in your health and fitness journey. Remember, it is a continuous process, and with dedication, perseverance, and a commitment to self-care, you can lead a healthier and more fulfilling life.

Encouragement to embark on a lifelong journey of health and fitness

Embarking on a journey of health and fitness is not just a short-term endeavor; it is a lifelong commitment to your well-being. As you have explored the various chapters and topics in this book, you have gained valuable knowledge and practical strategies to guide you on your path. Now, let us provide you with some encouragement as you embark on this lifelong journey:

Believe in Yourself:

You possess the inner strength and determination to achieve your health and fitness goals. Believe in yourself and your ability to make positive changes in your life. Remember, small steps taken consistently over time lead to significant transformations.

Embrace the Process:

Embrace the journey itself, not just the end goal. Enjoy the progress you make along the way and the positive changes you experience in your body, mind, and spirit. Celebrate every milestone, no matter how small, and appreciate the effort you put into improving your well-being.

Be Kind to Yourself:

Remember that health and fitness are about self-care, self-love, and self-improvement. Treat yourself with kindness and compassion, understanding that setbacks and challenges are part of the process. Be patient with yourself, and focus on progress rather than perfection.

Find Joy in Movement:

Discover activities that bring you joy and make you feel alive. Whether it's dancing, hiking, swimming, or practicing a sport, find ways to incorporate movement into your daily life that you genuinely enjoy. This will help you maintain a positive mindset and make fitness a sustainable part of your lifestyle.

Stay Consistent:

Consistency is the key to long-term success. Stay committed to your health and fitness goals, even during times when motivation may wane. Remember that every small effort counts and that consistent action over time yields powerful results.

Surround Yourself with Support:

Seek out a community of like-minded individuals who share your passion for health and fitness. Surround yourself with positive influences and find accountability partners who can motivate and inspire you on your journey. Together, you can overcome obstacles and celebrate achievements.

Embrace Balance:

Remember that health and fitness encompass not only physical well-being but also mental, emotional, and spiritual well-being. Strive for balance in all aspects of your life, ensuring that you prioritize self-care, rest, and recovery as much as you do exercise and nutrition.

Adapt and Evolve:

Your health and fitness journey will evolve as you grow and change. Embrace new challenges, explore different activities, and continue to expand your knowledge. Be open to trying new things and adjusting your approach as needed to sustain your progress and keep the journey exciting.

Enjoy the Benefits:

Embracing a lifestyle of health and fitness brings numerous benefits beyond physical changes. You will experience increased energy, improved mood, enhanced self-confidence, better sleep, reduced stress, and a greater sense of overall well-being. Embrace and appreciate these positive transformations.

Remember, this is not a quick fix or a temporary endeavor. It is a lifelong journey of self-improvement and self-care. Embrace the process, stay committed, and always prioritize your well-being. You have the power to shape your future and live a life filled with vitality and happiness. Now, go forth with determination, confidence, and excitement as you embark on this lifelong journey of health and fitness.

Resources for further exploration and support

As you continue your journey of health and fitness, it's important to have access to additional resources and support. Here are some suggestions for further exploration and finding support along the way:

Books and Literature:

There are numerous books available that delve deeper into specific aspects of health and fitness. Some highly recommended titles include "The Four-Hour Body" by Timothy Ferriss, "Atomic Habits" by James Clear, "The Mindful Athlete" by George Mumford, and "The Blue Zones" by Dan Buettner.

Online Communities and Forums:

Joining online communities and forums can provide a wealth of information and support. Websites like Reddit's r/Fitness and r/GetMotivated, Bodybuilding.com, and SparkPeople offer forums where you can connect with like-minded individuals, ask questions, and share experiences.

Fitness Apps and Trackers:

Utilize fitness apps and trackers to monitor your progress, track your workouts, and receive guidance. Popular apps like MyFitnessPal, Fitbit, and Strava offer features to help you set goals, track your nutrition, and connect with a community of fitness enthusiasts.

Professional Guidance:

Consider seeking professional guidance from certified personal trainers, nutritionists, or health coaches. They can provide personalized advice, create customized workout plans, and offer expert support tailored to your specific needs and goals.

Online Courses and Webinars:

Explore online courses and webinars offered by fitness professionals and reputable organizations. Platforms like Udemy, Coursera, and The Great Courses provide a wide range of health and fitness-related courses that you can take at your own pace.

Podcasts:

Podcasts are a great way to learn from experts and stay motivated. Some popular health and fitness podcasts include "The Model Health Show" by Shawn Stevenson, "The

Jillian Michaels Show," and "The Rich Roll Podcast." These podcasts cover various topics related to health, fitness, nutrition, and mindset.

Local Fitness Centers and Gyms:

Joining a local fitness center or gym can provide access to professional trainers, group classes, and a supportive community. Engaging with others who share similar goals can keep you motivated and provide a sense of camaraderie.

Wellness Retreats and Workshops:

Consider attending wellness retreats or workshops focused on health, fitness, mindfulness, and nutrition. These events offer immersive experiences and expert guidance to help you deepen your understanding and practice in various aspects of well-being.

Social Media Influencers and Bloggers:

Follow reputable health and fitness influencers and bloggers on social media platforms such as Instagram and YouTube. They often share tips, workouts, recipes, and motivational content that can inspire and educate you.

Remember, it's essential to critically evaluate the sources you encounter and seek evidence-based information from reputable professionals. Everyone's journey is unique, so choose resources and support systems that align with your personal values and goals.

By leveraging these resources and finding the support you need, you can continue to expand your knowledge, stay motivated, and make informed decisions on your health and fitness journey.